The
Assessment of Aphasia
and Related Disorders

The
Assessment of Aphasia
and Related Disorders

HAROLD GOODGLASS, Ph.D.

with the collaboration of
EDITH KAPLAN, Ph.D.

Boston Veterans Administration Hospital
and
Aphasia Research Center, Department of Neurology,
Boston University

LEA & FEBIGER   •   *Philadelphia*

Reprinted, 1976

ISBN 0–8121–0357–2

Published in Great Britain by Henry Kimpton Publishers, London

Library of Congress Catalog Card Number: 73–152024
Printed in the United States of America

Print Number: 5   4   3

PREFACE

World War II marked the beginning of a reawakening of interest in aphasia which has continued unabated until now. The immediate stimuli for this interest were the presence of large numbers of brain-injured, speech-disabled soldiers and the social obligation to rehabilitate them. Immediately on the heels of the postwar era came the burgeoning of activities related to the rehabilitation of the handicapped—particularly victims of stroke and head injury, of whom the aphasics make up an important segment. In response to this growth, the training of speech clinicians increased tremendously and, concurrently, the neuropsychological study of normal and pathological brain function attracted many able researchers.

A further and predictable response to these circumstances was the appearance on the market of a number of manuals on aphasia and aphasia testing. The earliest and most widely used was Eisenson's *Examining for Aphasia* (1954), followed by the Wepman and Jones *Language Modalities Test for Aphasia* (1961) and Schuell's *Differential Diagnosis of Aphasia with the Minnesota Test* (1965). In the area of childhood language disturbances, the McCarthy and Kirk *Illinois Test of Psycholinguistic Abilities* (1966) met wide acceptance.

Why, then, the need for another manual and test for aphasia? The principal answer is that the authors of the present work believe it offers features which give the examiner more insight into the patient's functioning and which serve as a bridge to relating test scores to the common aphasic syndromes recognized by neurologists. The Boston Diagnostic Aphasia Test was developed in a center where the rehabilitation of aphasics is part of a multidisciplinary approach, along with the study of the neuropathological correlates of the varieties of aphasia and the psycholinguistic analysis of aphasic language. The test inevitably reflects the converging interests of these disciplines.

The opening two chapters of the manual present the authors' orientation to the nature of aphasic disorders and the goals and rationale of the assessment procedure. While an effort is made to place this discussion in the context of the history and relevant current research on aphasia, it is by no means intended as a comprehensive review of either history or research. The third chapter cites the statistical data available up to the present time. Chapter 4 describes the test procedure, subtest by subtest, and is intended to serve as an instruction manual for the examiner. Chapter 5 describes additional, unstandardized, special language testing procedures, some of which are being investigated experimentally and others which are used informally at the center. Chapter 6 describes a supplementary nonverbal battery covering apraxia and the quantitative, visuospatial and somatognosic problems which, in addition to language, are so often implicated.

Finally, Chapter 7 describes the major aphasic syndromes as well as some of the rare "pure" forms of selective aphasia and shows how each pattern is reflected in the Aphasia Test score profile, with the help of selected case summaries.

This test and manual owe their existence primarily to the financial support and clinical facilities of the Boston Veterans Administration Hospital, particularly of the Aphasia Research Center. Support has also been received from NINDS Grants 07615 to Clark University and 06209 to Boston University, the latter being responsible for the establishment of the Boston University Aphasia Research Center. The authors' theoretical orientation has been influenced by Dr. Fred A. Quadfasel and Dr. Norman Geschwind during their respective tenures as Chief of Neurology at the Boston Veterans Administration Hospital. We are also indebted to Dr. Geschwind for his critical reading of the manuscript. Much of the testing was carried out by Miss Betty North and Mrs. Barbara Klein Efron. Some of the test items were developed with the assistance of Mr. Robert Sparks, Supervisor of Aphasia Therapy at the Boston Veterans Administration Hospital. Finally, we would like to acknowledge our patient and conscientious secretary, Gladys Bernardinelli, who saw us through many versions of both test and manuscript.

HAROLD GOODGLASS, PH.D.
EDITH KAPLAN, PH.D.
Boston, Massachusetts

CONTENTS

Page

Chapter 1. BACKGROUND 1

Chapter 2. THE NATURE OF THE DEFICITS 5

Chapter 3. STATISTICAL BACKGROUND . . 12

Chapter 4. TEST PROCEDURES AND RATIO-
NALE: MANUAL FOR THE BOS-
TON DIAGNOSTIC APHASIA TEST 24

Chapter 5. SUPPLEMENTARY LANGUAGE
TESTS 41

Chapter 6. SUPPLEMENTARY NON-
LANGUAGE TESTS 45

Chapter 7. MAJOR APHASIC SYNDROMES
AND ILLUSTRATIONS OF TEST
PATTERNS 54

REFERENCES 79

Chapter 1

BACKGROUND

The modern history of aphasia is usually dated back to the ferment over Broca's presentation of evidence for the localization of motor aphasia in the *Bulletin de la Société d'anthropologie* in 1861. However, the phenomenon of loss of speech due to brain injury is as old as recorded medicine and Benton's review (1964) establishes that virtually all of the currently recognized aphasic symptoms were described long before the nineteenth century. The three decades preceding Broca's historic contribution witnessed increasing interest and controversy over the mechanisms of organic language disorders (Hécaen and Dubois, 1969), so that the events of 1861 fell on fertile ground.

It was only with the work of Broca, Wernicke and their contemporaries, however, that certain organic impairments of language functions were finally grouped together under the term "aphasia," and recognized as distinct from the other intellectual impairments which might accompany them as by-products of cerebral damage. The almost exclusive association of language loss with injury to a portion of the left cerebral hemisphere was recognized during the 1860's and the concept of unilateral cerebral dominance thus arose. Moreover, within a few decades of Broca's first localizing discoveries, it became clear that certain specific patterns of language loss could reliably be assigned to lesions in specific regions *within* the language area. The fascinating history of these discoveries and the nineteenth-century theories about the neurological organization of language are reported in the classical works by Head (1926), Weisenburg and McBride (1935) and recent historical papers by Benton (1964) and Geschwind (1966).

The examination protocols of these neurologists, as detailed in their clinical reports, often reveal thorough inventories of language performance in all modalities. Moreover, since these workers were often sophisticated in problems of language, they paid attention to many of the more subtle aspects of aphasic language disorders and included analysis of grammar and syntax in their case studies.

In this presentation, we propose to continue in the tradition of approaching the aphasia examination as a psychological analysis and measurement of language-related skills on one hand, and on the other, as a problem in relating particular configurations of symptoms with their neuropathological correlates.

THE PURPOSES OF APHASIA TESTING

The examination for aphasia may be geared to any one of three general aims: (1) diagnosis of presence and type of aphasic syndrome, leading to inferences concerning cerebral localization; (2) measurement of the level of performance over a wide range, for both initial determination and detection of change over time; (3) comprehensive assessment of the assets and liabilities of the patient in all language areas as a guide to therapy.

It is possible to design tests which perform any one of these functions well but fall short in one or both of the others. The present test is designed to meet all three of these applications, making it maximally useful to the neurologist, the psychologist, the speech pathologist and the speech therapist.

The diagnostic aim is met by sampling, in as pure a form as possible, all the components of language which have proven useful in identifying aphasic syndromes; for instance, seriatim speech, repetition and performance with special word categories, such as right-left discrimination, body parts, colors, letters of the alphabet. Further, by means of rating scales and error classification, the examiner is directed to those features of language which are not readily reduced to pass-fail scores, but which are of critical importance in arriving at a diagnostic decision. These include speech melody, fluency, anomia, syntactic organization and the various forms of paraphasia.

The measurement function embodies certain requirements which are met in this test. These requirements are: (1) wide range of difficulty, (2) adequate subtest length for reliability and for discrimination of change and (3) standardization to provide an external reference point of degrees of severity in each area tested.

The survey of the aphasic patient's assets and liabilities is made by comparing the effectiveness of various alternative ways of eliciting speech, comprehension, reading and writing. Not only is the survey exceptionally complete, but the availability of standardized scores in each subtest frees the examiner from purely impressionistic judgments about the patient's relative impairment in one area as compared to another.

Limitations

The limitations of this test battery are those which are inherent in any aphasia test. The materials and procedures provided by the test merely serve as convenient aids for sampling relevant performances of the patient. The scores do not objectively and automatically classify the patient nor point

to the optimum approach to therapy. The greater the experience of the examiner, the more useful the interpretations that can be made from the test record. The case illustrations will serve as a guide but not as a source of cookbook formulas for diagnosis.

PRINCIPLES UNDERLYING THIS EXAMINATION

The design of this Aphasia Test is based on the observation that various components of language may be selectively damaged by aphasia and that this selectivity is a clue to (1) the anatomical organization of language in the brain, (2) the localization of the causative lesion and (3) the functional interactions (e.g., inhibitory, regulatory, selective) of various parts of the language system.

It must be pointed out that the foregoing position is not universally accepted. Schuell, Jenkins and Jiménez-Pabón (1964), for example, attribute most of the significant variations among aphasia subtests to impairment of general language capacity. There are many factors in the aphasia testing situation which tend to erase the evidence for any underlying independence of components in language:

1. It is difficult to devise a single task which can be passed or failed through only one process.

2. Though the various neural subsystems of language may be selectively vulnerable at certain anatomical points, they are almost certainly intermingled in other areas of the cortex. The larger the lesion in these areas, the greater the effect on many functions.

3. The bulk of the clinical material for quantitative studies comes from cases in which large lesions are the rule, implicating, simultaneously, functionally diverse areas. Small lesions producing isolated disorders occur less frequently and therefore have a smaller

effect in any study which groups all cases together.

4. The usual distribution of severity of aphasics in hospitals, as Schuell points out, is bimodal, with many severe and residual aphasics but few at intermediate levels. This spread overemphasizes the severity factor, producing large intercorrelations and obscuring differences in process between tasks.

If all language performance in aphasia were merely a function of the status of "general language ability," the ideal aphasia test would consist of a handful of tasks most highly loaded in this factor, which would be presumed to predict fairly well the standing on all other tests. Alternatively, we might settle for a general communication score. We accept the usefulness of these global measures, but hold that there is also much more to be learned from an aphasia examination.

Returning to the construction of the present test, we tried first to assess the components of language as nearly as possible in isolated form. It is impossible to reach this ideal completely since one can test an expressive function only by choosing some instrumental input channel through which to elicit the expressive behavior. In the same way, one can test receptive functions only by designating an instrumental response modality through which the subject demonstrates his comprehension. Generally, we regard the instrumental modality as only one of several possible "windows" on the capacity in question. If the validity of the view through one "window" is in doubt, we improvise another, if it is not already provided by the test. We specifically reject the view of language as being based primarily on a collection of stimulus-response systems. In this respect, our approach is different from that of Wepman's *Language Modalities Test for Aphasia* (1961).

For example, desiring to know how a patient appreciates oral spelling, we choose the response mode or "window" of having him tell us orally what we have spelled for him. If his speech production is much impaired, it provides a clouded "window" and we must find another approach to assess his comprehension of orally spelled words— perhaps multiple-choice selection of pictures to correspond with the spelled word (not provided in the test). To take another example, if we wish to test the word-finding ability of a patient, we may approach it through the instrumental mode of showing him objects visually, we may have him feel them tactually or listen to the sounds they make or answer questions requiring their names. Each of these "windows" on word-finding has its own characteristics as a receptive modality which make it more or less effective as a means of eliciting the desired response. Studies by Spreen, Benton and Van Allen (1966) and by Goodglass, Barton and Kaplan (1968) show that, with few exceptions, aphasics name objects equally well through whatever sensory modality they are presented. The concept of independent stimulus-response channels going directly from each modality-specific receptive system to the oral output system is not supported. The few instances of modality-specific naming defects are of great interest, but where anatomic information is available, it indicates isolation of the sensory input from the entire left cerebral language system.

In playing down the role of stimulus-response units in language, we argue that the vast bulk of functional language behavior involves either self-initiated linguistic output or responses in which it is apparent that complex intermediary steps have occurred between the perception of a linguistic or other sensory input and the output. The immediate response to a linguistic stimulus is an implicit one which we can only assess indirectly through the test performance which we choose. However, there are a number of elementary language skills which do not require comprehension or formulation of a meaningful message and which may be defended as stimulus-response units. These are, for the most part, direct imitations of the input, as in the case of repetition of spoken language or copying of written language. Even in these cases, we must assure ourselves that the receptive process and the output capability are intact before considering a performance failure to be a loss of the stimulus-response unit. For example, it may be shown that oral repetition can break down in the presence of intact auditory comprehension and considerable fluency of spontaneous or conversational speech.

Can the same be said for copying written language, in cases where copying is the only means of eliciting a patient's writing? In most cases—especially when the patient can transcribe—we are probably dealing with a direct evocation of writing movements in response to seeing letters. When all means of recalling writing have been lost, the patient may still copy slavishly, but he is now calling on his general ability to reproduce simple geometrical forms.

In summary, then, the subtests of the battery in most cases represent alternative "windows" which enable us to infer the status of an underlying capacity. In a few cases, they are direct samples of a stimulus-response unit which usually represents one of the elementary language performance skills.

Chapter 2

THE NATURE OF THE DEFICITS

Normal language may be regarded as depending on a complex interaction between sensory-motor skills, symbolic associations and habituated syntactic patterns, all at the service of the speaker's intent to communicate, and subject to the intellectual capacity which he brings to the task of manipulating them so as to carry out his intent. Aphasia refers to the disturbance of any or all of the skills, association and habits of spoken or written language, produced by injury to certain brain areas which are specialized for these functions. Disturbances of language usage which are due to paralysis or incoordination of the musculature of speech or writing or to poor vision or hearing or to severe intellectual impairment are not, by themselves, aphasic. Such disorders may accompany an aphasia and thus complicate the clinical manifestations of the language defect proper.

A century of intensive analysis of aphasic symptoms has produced considerable agreement as to the component deficits, some of which may appear in nearly pure form, or may stand out by their severity on a background of milder impairment in the remaining language skills. Thus, one may find extreme, selective disorders of auditory comprehension, object-naming, articulation, reading or repetition, to give a few instances. Not only is there wide consensus as to the individual component deficits to be observed, but the common clusters of defects (i.e., the major aphasic syndromes) emerge repeatedly in the interpretive observations of dozens of careful writers, though often under different names based on different theoretical biases.

The deficits of aphasia and their common clustering cannot, in general, be deduced by a logical analysis of the normal speech process; they are empirically derived. The subtests of this aphasia battery have, in turn, been chosen so as to elicit quantitive evidence of the many possible specific areas of deficit. Where objective quantification is not feasible, the examiner is provided with rating scales.

ENUMERATION OF AREAS OF DEFICIT

Articulation

Patients with the most severe articulatory disorders are unable voluntarily to produce simple sounds even by imitation. Each effort may end up with the emission of the same, recurrent word or nonsense syllable, to the chagrin of the patient. In somewhat milder form, the patient may be considerably aided by imitation, but articulate laboriously, with distortions of the more difficult sounds, particularly consonant blends. Vowels tend to return to normal earlier than do consonants. Success in finding the articulatory movement sequences for a given word is often an all-or-none affair. That is, as the patient improves, he may pronounce common words and phrases normally, but experience severe articulatory difficulty with less common words.

Articulatory difficulty, as an aphasic component, is distinguished from nonaphasic dysarthria by its variability. The aphasic often reveals perfectly normal articulation during automatized sequences (counting) or in repeating or during exclamations. Increased effort may only aggravate his difficulty. A nonaphasic dysarthria is more constant under all conditions and may be somewhat controlled by attention and effort on the patient's part.

Because the task of repetition often masks the articulatory difficulty of aphasics, this standard approach to testing articulation is not used here. Instead, the present examination relies on articulation ratings for each response in a variety of speech tasks, as well as on an articulation rating scale.

Loss of Verbal Fluency

The ability to produce words in connected sequences is closely associated with ease of articulation, but is not *always* predicted by articulation. That is, patients who pronounce individual words clearly may go through a separate effort to emit each word or, at best, produce very short word groupings with each separate effort. More rarely, poor articulation may be compatible with considerable fluency. Fluency is best rated in terms of the longest occasional uninterrupted strings of words which are produced. It has been found to be reliably ratable in this way and to be an important diagnostic criterion (Goodglass, Quadfasel and Timberlake, 1964).

Fluency is best judged from speech production during extended conversation and free narrative. The present examination procedure prescribes an interview, followed by presentation of a picture situation as a stimulus for a short narrative description. A rating scale for fluency is included in a set of six rating scales for those speech characteristics which are difficult to quantify objectively.

Word-finding Difficulty

Virtually all aphasics suffer some restriction in the repertory of words which they have available for speech and require in-creased time to produce these words. For most patients, the frequent words of the language are the first recovered and are produced with the briefest delay. In some patients, however, loss of the power to evoke words corresponding to specific concepts is disproportionately severe as compared to the level of fluency and articulation. These patients show a striking inability to name even common objects, action words, colors, adjectives and other categories of words. There is a subtle qualitative difference between the general restriction of vocabulary, common to most aphasics, and the selective loss of the ability to evoke specific words, which is called "word-finding difficulty" or "anomia."

Since patients with anomia are usually relatively fluent in producing a flow of small talk or rambling uninformative speech, it has been noted that their speech sounds "empty," that is, lacking in the critical words necessary to convey meaning.

The obvious way of testing word-finding difficulty would seem to be to present pictures or questions requiring the selection of a particular word in response. However, this test approach, by itself, fails to distinguish the anomic patient from the patient who cannot articulate or from the patient with a generalized severe restriction of speech. One of the common features of anomia is the selectivity shown among categories of words. Nouns are the most severely impaired category, while many patients retain their ability to name letters and numbers (Goodglass, Klein, Carey and Jones, 1966). We have, therefore, made a special point of sampling each of several word categories.

The decision as to whether word-finding difficulty is a significant feature of an aphasic's speech pattern, however, cannot be made from a correctness count on any single test but rather depends on the pattern observed in conversation. Here again, we provide a rating scale to be applied to the sample of conversation and narrative speech.

Repetition

The ability to reproduce, from aural presentation, patterns of familiar speech sound is normally acquired early in life and is one of the most elementary mechanisms at the core of spoken language. Mental defectives who have little capacity to convey or understand information through language may have this particular sensory-motor system intact, so that they can echo speech and can acquire passages by rote.

Repetition in aphasia may be disturbed at three points in the process. First, the patient may fail at the level of recognition. He may fail to grasp the sounds as words and, consequently, refuse to attempt to repeat them, or he may capture only certain fragments of the spoken model. Second, he may fail at the level of articulation in spite of his ability to demonstrate that he knows the meaning of the test words or sentence. Finally, he may fail because of a selective dissociation between auditory input and the speech-output systems. The latter group of patients may demonstrate fairly fluent speech and near-perfect comprehension, yet have extraordinary difficulty in repeating what they have heard. This difficulty is increased by the length and unfamiliarity of the material to be repeated. In this aphasia examination, tests for repetition of words as well as for sentences of increasing length are included.

Not only is the selective impairment of repetition diagnostically significant, but also its selective retention in an otherwise very severe aphasia.

Seriatim Speech

It has long been observed that the reciting of memorized sequences (e.g. counting, days of the week) may be partially spared in severely aphasic patients of all types. Thus, while these items are almost always included in aphasia tests, they rarely are diagnostically important for distinguishing between varieties of aphasics. An occasional patient who may

otherwise be bereft of useful speech will show extraordinary retention of the ability to recite, not only the familiar word series, but even poetry or long prayers. This configuration is particularly notable when associated with good repetition. Like repetition, the ability to reel off a memorized sequence represents the operation of an elementary sensory-motor skill of spoken language which says nothing about the ability to associate meaning to the spoken word, either receptively or expressively.

In this aphasia examination, the performance of automatized speech is sampled through the usual tasks of reciting numbers, days, months and the alphabet, as well as nursery rhymes.

Loss of Grammar and Syntax

Gross clinical impression tells us that some aphasics are totally lacking in the ability to place words together in grammatically organized sequences, while other patients, no less disabled in effective speech, may have great facility in framing sentences of many varieties. Grammatical facility is usually associated with word-finding difficulty; grammatical impoverishment is associated with loss of fluency and is often accompanied by good word-finding.

Close examination of the problem of disturbed grammar reveals that several different elementary skills contribute to normal grammatical performance. Among these skills are:

Verbal retention span. The patient who can retain only a four- or five-syllable span cannot conceive a sentence plan running for a longer duration than his span and is forced to concentrate his thoughts into short utterances having primitive grammatical form.

Facility in initiating speech. Many aphasics cannot start an utterance with an unstressed word, but gravitate to the first stressed or salient word, such as the noun or principal verb. The result is that sentences which should begin with pronouns, prepositions or auxiliary verbs, lose their small grammatical words.

Discrimination of relational concepts. Certain grammatical errors appear to be due to a loss of the ability to discriminate, by the use of grammatical words and inflection, between such contrasts as present and future, masculine and feminine, before and after. This difficulty, when it is present, extends to the comprehension, as well as the expression, of these distinctions.

Knowledge of grammatical rules. The evidence from aphasia is that the grammatical intactness of speech is largely a function of retention of sequential verbal habits, rather than of the conscious application of rules. Loss of verbal fluency interrupts the sequence of cues which the aphasic needs to proceed with syntactically correct sentences. When a patient is intellectually intact, however, he may compensate with his conscious knowledge of the rules of sentence structure and overcome the handicap of laborious, interrupted speech. Specific rules for at least a small repertory of constructions may also be taught.

The objective testing of the components of grammatical performance is still in the experimental stage. Because of their diverse underlying causes, we do not consider the combined tabulation of grammatical errors very informative. Recognizing the descriptive value of grammatical facility, however, we provide a rating scale for a judgment of the variety of syntactical forms available in the patient's speech.

Paraphasia

Paraphasia refers to the production of unintended syllables, words or phrases during the effort to speak. In general, paraphasia is characteristic of patients whose speech sounds are fluently uttered. The distorted pronunciation of patients with poor articulation does *not* come under this heading.

Under the rubric of paraphasia, the following specific varieties are diagnostically distinctive:

Literal (or phonemic) paraphasia. In spite of easy articulation of individual sounds, the patient produces syllables in the wrong order or distorts his words with unintended sounds. For example, "pipe" may become "Hike . . . no, pike . . . pipe!" Some phonemic features (usually the vowels and the number of syllables) of the intended words are preserved, thus distinguishing literal paraphasic utterances from paraphasic *jargon*. When words are grossly distorted with literal paraphasia, we use the term *neologistic distortion*, an extreme literal paraphasic error.

Verbal paraphasia. When an unintended word is inadvertently used in place of another, the substituted words are usually related in connotative sphere (e.g., "my mother" in place of "my wife") to the intended word. These may be referred to as "semantic paraphasias" as opposed to "random paraphasia" where the substitution seems totally capricious, or as opposed to "perseverative paraphasia" where the word used crops up again from something said just previously. Verbal paraphasias, which are *unintended*, should be distinguished from "one-word circumlocutions" in which the patient deliberately chooses an approximation to his intended idea because of his word-finding difficulty (e.g., he substitutes the word, "Chesterfield," for "cigarette").

Extended jargon. This applies to running speech (phrases or sentences) which includes senseless words or neologisms. An important characteristic of this speech is that it is produced uncritically. One may include in this category repetitious, extremely circumlocutory speech which is devoid of content.

Scoring of paraphasia. In this examination, each instance of paraphasia is tallied as it occurs during the testing. Separate columns are provided for literal, neologistic, verbal and extended paraphasia. The relative frequency of the various types of paraphasia is reflected in the z-score profile sheet. In addition, the occurrence of paraphasia in running speech is rated on the Profile of Speech Characteristics.

Auditory Comprehension

Disturbances of auditory comprehension may take various forms, with varying degrees of severity in each aspect. The present battery measures some, but not all, of these dimensions. For example, a most dramatic, but uncommon, form of comprehension defect is "word-deafness" in which the patient reacts *as though* he has not heard the words spoken to him or has captured only fragments of their sounds. On repeated presentation, he may succeed in grasping the sounds and then, at once, understand the word. More commonly (as seen in Wernicke's aphasia), the defect does not involve the recognition of sounds, but rather the association of meaning to them, for the patient may repeat aloud, uncomprehendingly, words spoken to him. While both these forms of disorder may produce the same objective test score, their clinical manifestations are clearly different.

In particular, Wernicke's aphasics are often strikingly worse in grasping words in isolation than in a sentence context. They benefit from the additional clues to meaning which they garner from the rest of the sentence. Thus, length of utterance does not increase difficulty of comprehension in a simple linear fashion. It is only when length is combined with the demand to grasp multiple significant informational elements that comprehension suffers.

When auditory comprehension is only partially impaired, the patient's success may depend on the familiarity of the words used, on the length and informational density of the message and on the intellectual simplicity of the message to be understood. In this battery, we examine for *comprehension vocabulary* by means of a "word-discrimination" subtest of single words; we examine capacity for information by means of commands of increasing length; we examine intellectual grasp by means of a set of "yes"-"no" questions demanding increasing powers of inference about questions of fact, but not beyond the capacity of average adults.

Further, recognizing that words of a given semantic class may be selectively affected, we divide the word-discrimination test into "objects," "actions," "colors," "numbers," "letters," "geometric shapes" and "body parts." We have not incorporated a separate section of whole body commands (e.g., "Stand up, turn around, walk backwards and return to your seat"). Paradoxically, these are often well preserved.

Currently under study is the difficulty of grasping certain grammatical words and grammatical constructions, such as prepositional relationships and instances where meaning depends on word order (e.g., "my brother's wife" vs. "my wife's brother"). These may be severely impaired in patients who have excellent word discrimination, yet unaccountably fail to grasp certain commands. Thus, the present battery does not deprive the examiner of the opportunity to improvise and explore the patient's capacity. The examiner must take into account the easy fatigability of comprehension, failures brought about by difficulty in shifting between topics and the facilitating effect of making the conversation personally relevant to the patient.

Reading

The normal acquisition of reading appears to be based on the prior mastery of auditory language. Most readers will report having an inner auditory experience in the course of silent reading. In the experimental laboratory, MacKay (1968) has shown that misspellings phonetically different from the correct word are perceived more accurately than those having the same phonetic value as the correct word. Evidence from aphasia supports the concept that the neurological basis of reading includes the auditory comprehension system, in addition to structures which provide an association between the auditory and the visual processes. Thus, aphasias involving severe impairment of auditory language almost invariably impair reading—particularly reading of connected material. The most striking apparent exception to this rule is in the case of pure word-deafness (described above), where reading is preserved. The anatomic reason proposed for this exception is that the auditory association area is essentially intact, but disconnected from its input from the primary auditory areas.

The relation between reading and auditory comprehension levels is often confusing in the Wernicke's aphasic. These patients, as we have observed, may fail to grasp a word spoken to them out of context, even while repeating it correctly. On seeing the same word written, they often understand it at once. Thus, at the one-word level, reading is superior to auditory comprehension. When the written message increases to sentence length, its difficulty increases enormously, while comprehension of the spoken message is sometimes facilitated by the sentence context.

May not reading comprehension be autonomous from the auditory comprehension system? We know that deaf-mutes learn to read and grasp meaning without ever having had an auditory experience of the word. It is plausible that this mode of reading plays at least a secondary role in normal reading, as well. Supporting evidence shows that some aphasics grasp meaning while saying the wrong word aloud. Conversely, some patients will point to a written word related in meaning, but not in sound, to a spoken model.

The analytic examination of reading requires determination of whether letters and words are recognized as familiar configurations, quite apart from their meaning. Can spoken and written words be matched on the basis of phonic associations, still without concern for meaning? Both of these functions are examined by means of multiple-choice subtests. In the rare cases of alexia caused purely by disconnection of the visual input from the cortical language area, the

patient continues to understand oral spelling. Comprehension of oral spelling may be lost either because of impaired recognition or limited auditory span for letter names or because of disturbance of the audio-visual associations on which reading is based.

The simplest level of reading for meaning is that of pairing written words with corresponding concepts, usually in the form of pictures. In the present examination, a multiple-choice selection of pictures is used. Comprehension of connected text is then tested by means of a graded series of multiple-choice sentence completion items, increasing from three-word sentence to paragraph length.

Writing

Writing is the most complex of the language modalities and has a correspondingly large number of dimensions for examination. At the level of mere motor execution, writing may fail with respect to the recall of the form of letters or of the movements involved in producing them. As in speech, there are automatized, serial tasks such as one's name and address, or the alphabet, which may be preserved when all other writing is lost. Slavish copying from a printed model may still be possible when the subject cannot transcribe into cursive script.

While, in the speaker's mind, the smallest significant units of oral speech are morphemes, when we deal with writing, letters have much more autonomy. The recall of letters to dictation is, therefore, tested prior to examining the ability to write words to dictation.

When a word is written to dictation, we do not know whether the process involved is primarily one of phonetic translation from sound to spelling or whether comprehension of the meaning of the word has played an intermediary role. However, when the patient is required to write the names of pictured objects, we know that the initiating process is the concept of the object and we are testing "written word-finding." Observation of the writing process and of patient's errors indicate that three types of association are at work. One is the automatic translation of sounds into the motor sequences for letters, following the phonic rules of the language; another is the recall of syllables and short words as complete graphic motor sequences, bolstered by a visual model of the word configurations; a third is the availability of oral spelling as a guide to writing. Because oral spelling is unhampered by the slowness of recalling and writing individual letters, we often find oral spelling a bit superior to written spelling to dictation. Only by specifically testing each process do we obtain an inkling as to how they are interacting in the patient's performance of a complex writing task.

As we raised the question about reading, we may ask how independent written expression is from formulated oral language. Is there a direct association between concept and written expression that does not go through the intermediary of auditorily formulated inner speech? The performance of aphasics indicates such autonomous writing may occur at the one-word level, when, for example, a patient writes or spells orally a word which he cannot recall in speech. Further evidence is seen in patients who, on dictation of a given word, write another which is related in meaning, but not in sound (paragraphia). However, the vast preponderance of aphasic performance indicates that writing is built on the capacity to formulate spoken language. Thus, the ability to write may approach, but rarely exceed, the capacity to speak. As in the case of reading, the exception to this rule is in patients whose disorder is purely articulatory and apparently spares the speech formulation system.

The medium of writing does not provide the melodic and rhythmic sentence contour which helps the aphasic to organize his grammatical sequences and, particularly, to fit in the small connectives and inflectional forms. Because writing is a slower, word-by-word process, sentence-writing makes a heavy demand on knowledge of grammatical rules and on retention of the string of projected words, along with recall of what has already been written. Consequently, grammar may be more primitive in written language than in speech.

In the present aphasia battery, the writing of connected material is elicited by dictation and by presentation of a story-picture which the patient is asked to describe in writing.

Chapter 3

STATISTICAL BACKGROUND

An evaluation of the reliability of the subtests was undertaken by selecting protocols of thirty-four patients who were distributed as follows on degree of severity of aphasia.

N	Level	Description
0	0	No communication possible.
11	1	Communication possible only by examiner's questioning and guessing.
6	2	Patient carries share of conversation but range of information exchanged is limited.
7	3	Speech is defective in form and content but patient can convey almost all ideas.
6	4	Obvious handicap is present although speech is largely correct and there is no limitation on expression.
4	5	Residual aphasia with only subjective difficulties.

The Kuder-Richardson method of determining subtest reliability was applied. The resulting reliability coefficients are listed in Table 1. The subtests for which reliability data are omitted are those which are not based on a series of scoreable items, hence, not appropriate for this reliability measure.

The reliability coefficients obtained indicate good internal consistency within subtests with respect to what the items are measuring. Reliability, in the sense of repeatability of results on retesting any patient, varies among aphasics to a degree rarely found in other types of patients. Some subjects have wide fluctuations in efficiency from day to day as well as fluctuations depending on time of day. Once recovery has stabilized, however, the majority of aphasics will, on retest, repeat their original performance fairly closely. Test-retest data have not been obtained with this instrument.

Table 1. Reliability Coefficients of Subtests

	r_{xx}
Auditory Comprehension	
Word Discrimination	.96
Body-part Identification	.68
Commands	.91
Complex Ideational Material	.89
Oral Expression	
Oral Agility—Nonverbal	.83
Oral Agility—Verbal	.89
Automatized Sequences	.82
Repetition of Words	.92
Repetition of Phrases	
a. High Probability	.90
b. Low Probability	.91
Word-reading	.95
Responsive Naming	.92
Visual Confrontation Naming	.98
Oral Sentence-reading	.94
Understanding Written Language	
Symbol and Word Discrimination	.90
Phonetic Association	
a. Word Recognition	.80
b. Comprehension of Oral Spelling	.91
Word-picture Matching	.92
Reading Sentences and Paragraphs	.90
Writing	
Spelling to Dictation	.89
Written Confrontation Naming	.92

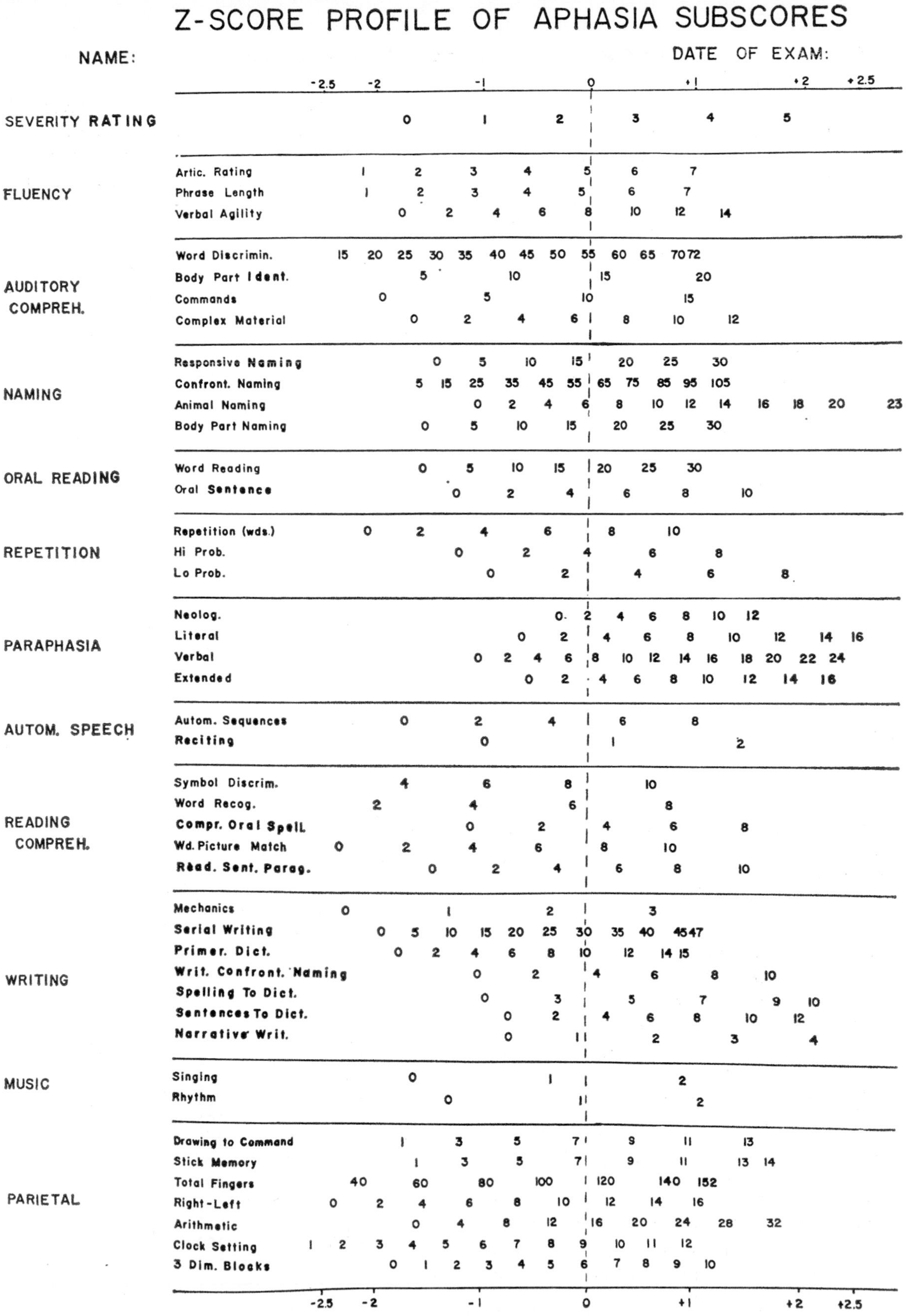

Z-SCORE PROFILE OF APHASIA SUBSCORES

NAME: DATE OF EXAM:

Scale: -2.5   -2   -1   0   +1   +2   +2.5

SEVERITY RATING
- 0   1   2   3   4   5

FLUENCY
- Artic. Rating: 1   2   3   4   5   6   7
- Phrase Length: 1   2   3   4   5   6   7
- Verbal Agility: 0   2   4   6   8   10   12   14

AUDITORY COMPREH.
- Word Discrimin.: 15   20   25   30   35   40   45   50   55   60   65   70 72
- Body Part Ident.: 5   10   15   20
- Commands: 0   5   10   15
- Complex Material: 0   2   4   6   8   10   12

NAMING
- Responsive Naming: 0   5   10   15   20   25   30
- Confront. Naming: 5   15   25   35   45   55   65   75   85   95   105
- Animal Naming: 0   2   4   6   8   10   12   14   16   18   20   23
- Body Part Naming: 0   5   10   15   20   25   30

ORAL READING
- Word Reading: 0   5   10   15   20   25   30
- Oral Sentence: 0   2   4   6   8   10

REPETITION
- Repetition (wds.): 0   2   4   6   8   10
- Hi Prob.: 0   2   4   6   8
- Lo Prob.: 0   2   4   6   8

PARAPHASIA
- Neolog.: 0.   2   4   6   8   10   12
- Literal: 0   2   4   6   8   10   12   14   16
- Verbal: 0   2   4   6   8   10   12   14   16   18   20   22   24
- Extended: 0   2   4   6   8   10   12   14   16

AUTOM. SPEECH
- Autom. Sequences: 0   2   4   6   8
- Reciting: 0   1   2

READING COMPREH.
- Symbol Discrim.: 4   6   8   10
- Word Recog.: 2   4   6   8
- Compr. Oral Spell: 0   2   4   6   8
- Wd. Picture Match: 0   2   4   6   8   10
- Read. Sent. Parag.: 0   2   4   6   8   10

WRITING
- Mechanics: 0   1   2   3
- Serial Writing: 0   5   10   15   20   25   30   35   40   45 47
- Primer. Dict.: 0   2   4   6   8   10   12   14 15
- Writ. Confront. Naming: 0   2   4   6   8   10
- Spelling To Dict.: 0   3   5   7   9   10
- Sentences To Dict.: 0   2   4   6   8   10   12
- Narrative Writ.: 0   1   2   3   4

MUSIC
- Singing: 0   1   2
- Rhythm: 0   2

PARIETAL
- Drawing to Command: 1   3   5   7   9   11   13
- Stick Memory: 1   3   5   7   9   11   13   14
- Total Fingers: 40   60   80   100   120   140   152
- Right-Left: 0   2   4   6   8   10   12   14   16
- Arithmetic: 0   4   8   12   16   20   24   28   32
- Clock Setting: 1   2   3   4   5   6   7   8   9   10   11   12
- 3 Dim. Blocks: 0   1   2   3   4   5   6   7   8   9   10

Scale: -2.5   -2   -1   0   +1   +2   +2.5

FIGURE 1.   Z-score profile of aphasia subscores.

STANDARDIZATION

The classification of any aphasic symptom configuration depends on the relative preservation of performance in various areas. Subtests covering these various areas vary in length and in absolute level of difficulty. Only the most experienced clinician can have any confidence in judging relative degrees of impairment between, for example, a score on a ten-item written spelling test and a score on a thirty-six-item picture-naming test. Thus it was important to develop some method of weighting so as to make subtest scores comparable among themselves.

The basic methodological problem is that one cannot be sure of the significance of a mean score for aphasics on any test because the distribution of degrees of severity of aphasia is not known and may be highly skewed. Since we have access only to that part of the aphasic population which comes to the hospital and stays for rehabilitation, we have no way of knowing how they compare to the population of all aphasics.

In order to circumvent this problem, we decided to assign our aphasics to the six clinically defined severity levels listed on page 12 and compute subtest z-scores independently for patients at each severity level above the lowest. This procedure yielded five z-score subtest profile charts, the appropriate one to be chosen according to the patient's severity level. We felt that the cumbersomeness of this procedure would be justified if different profiles resulted from similar combinations of scores for patients at different severity levels.

Plotting of a number of patients' profiles on z-score charts based on severity groups other than their own did not significantly affect their profiles, other than to move them, intact, back or forth on the severity dimension. It was, therefore, decided that, for practical purposes, we could disregard the question of whether the distribution of our aphasic sample truly represented the population and proceed as though it did. The z-score profile chart presented in Figure 1 is based on data from 207 patients at severity levels 1 through 5. These z-scores are based on the range, mean and standard deviation of the patients on each subtest as outlined in Table 2.

Table 2. Range, Mean and Standard Deviation of Aphasics on Each Subtest

	N	Range	M	SD
Severity Rating	152	1–5	2.4	1.4
Articulation Rating	147	1–7	5.1	1.9
Phrase-length Rating	147	1–7	5.2	2.0
Paraphasia (Neologistic)	180	0–10	1.8	6.7
Paraphasia (Literal)	180	0–29	3.1	5.0
Paraphasia (Verbal)	180	0–35	7.4	7.2
Paraphasia (Extended)	180	0–43	3.2	5.9
Word Discrimination	194	2–72	55.6	17.4
Body-part Identification	195	0–20	14.2	5.8
Commands	193	0–15	10.2	5.2
Complex Ideational Material	192	0–12	6.6	4.0
Verbal Agility	191	0–14	8.1	4.6
Nonverbal Agility	183	0–12	5.2	3.1
Automatized Sequences	191	0–8	5.0	2.9
Reciting	186	0–2	0.8	0.8
Singing	183	0–2	1.3	0.8
Rhythm	186	0–2	1.0	0.8
Repetition of Words	192	0–10	7.3	3.3
High-probability Repetition	187	0–8	3.9	3.2
Low-probability Repetition	186	0–8	2.6	2.9
Word-reading	191	0–30	18.2	11.8
Responsive Naming	192	0–30	16.3	11.3
Visual Confrontation Naming	188	0–105	62.0	35.9
Body-part Naming	50	0–30	17.0	11.1
Animal-naming	183	0–35	6.3	60
Oral Sentence-reading	187	0–10	4.6	3.6
Symbol and Word Discrimination	193	0–10	8.5	2.6
Word Recognition	193	0–8	6.3	2.2
Comprehension of Oral Spelling	193	0–8	3.4	3.1
Word-picture Matching	192	0–10	7.5	3.2
Reading Sentences and Paragraphs	189	0–10	5.0	3.4
Writing Mechanics	191	0–3	2.3	1.0
Serial Writing	187	0–47	30.6	16.0
Primer-level Dictation	187	0–15	9.8	5.5
Spelling to Dictation	184	0–10	3.7	2.9
Written Confrontation Naming	182	0–10	3.7	3.5
Narrative Writing	180	0–4	1.1	1.4
Sentences to Dictation	177	0–12	3.2	4.4

CLUSTERING OF SUBTESTS

Two approaches were taken to evaluate the interrelationships among the functions tested in this battery. The first was an inspection of clusters appearing in an inter-correlation matrix of all the subtests. The second was a factor analysis. Included in both analyses were the subtests of the supplementary nonlanguage tests of spatial-quantitative-somatognosic tasks ('parietal lobe' battery) described in Chapter 6. The language tasks comprised thirty-eight variables and the nonlanguage task eleven more; all forty-nine are included in the intercorrelation matrix and the factor analyses. The subjects were 111 aphasics, 43 of whom had received the aphasia battery only; the remaining subjects received both the aphasia battery and the supplementary nonlanguage tests.

The clustering of subtests is a clue to what may be significant psychological components in the performance of aphasics. However, the presence or absence of these clusters must be interpreted with extreme caution because they are, in part, artifacts both of the patient population used and of the tests which were chosen for the battery. Moreover, once a pair of subtests is found to be correlated, the basis for the correlation may be either a common psychological factor or the anatomical contiguity of the brain areas affecting the two functions involved.

With respect to the effect of the sampling of patients, the emergence of independent performance factors depends on having a representation of patients with selective deficits of various kinds, some of which may be quite rare. Thus, in a population of patients with widespread vascular damage of varying severity, there will be widespread impairment in all language modalities, varying in intensity from patient to patient. Correlational analysis of their test scores will yield high intercorrelations among all language performances and factor analysis will yield an overwhelming first factor produced by degrees of severity. If we look no further than the mathematical surface, we can accept this as proof of a general language factor. Given the nature of lesions causing aphasia, we cannot help obtaining such a factor, unless the population is chosen to include only patients with highly selective deficits corresponding to well-circumscribed lesions. If, in the originally described population, we happened to have a patient with a case of pure word-deafness, the possibility of an independent auditory receptive factor would still be rejected mathematically, because the one case would hardly affect the correlations arising from the group as a whole. We are left with the unpalatable suggestion that, if we wish to demonstrate the factorial independence of aphasic symptoms, we must select a population in which a sufficient number of patients have each symptom in *relatively isolated* (not necessarily pure) form, or show some selectivity in the sparing of certain language functions. Although this smacks of circular reasoning and of data manipulation, it has more to recommend it than the undiscriminating accumulation of consecutive cases without concern for the makeup of the population.

The present sample has a greater proportion of selective aphasias than would have been the case if every patient coming through the unit, including all global aphasics, had been tested. Because of the impossibility of testing every patient, preference was given to those who were being prepared for case conference—namely those whose configuration of symptoms were of some interest. While this did not eliminate global aphasics, it did result in a sampling bias away from that group of patients—a bias which we believe is conducive to more meaningful results.

As an example of how the selection of subtest measures may affect the appearance of factors, we may consider the example of the present battery in which we have included rating-scale measures of articulation and phrase-length, along with paraphasia counts. These appear with strong positive loadings on Factor III, while tasks demanding auditory comprehension are negatively loaded on this factor. Without the first group of measures, we might have regarded Factor III as an "auditory comprehension deficit factor." With the data on hand, however, it seems more reasonable to consider it a "Wernicke's aphasia" factor, since the configuration of high fluency, paraphasia and impaired comprehension are the distinguishing features of Wernicke's aphasia. (See discussion of syndromes, Chapter 7.) In interpreting this factor, we would be unjustified in assuming a common psychological ability linking paraphasia, fluency and impaired comprehension. They may just as easily be linked by anatomical contiguity of the lesions determining these symptoms.

With these cautions in mind, we will consider the intercorrelations and factorial structure reflected in our test battery. Inspection of the intercorrelation matrix shows that most correlations of more than .50 occurred between tests which had in common one of the following features:

Paraphasia
Recital-repetition
Auditory Comprehension
Writing
Speech Fluency
Word-finding
Reading
Visual-spatial Somatognosic

Examining each of these clusters in succession, we find the following correlations between the subtests of each cluster and with tasks outside the defined cluster.

Within the paraphasia cluster:

	Literal	Verbal	Other
Neologistic	.26	.31	.28
Literal	——	.62	.38
Verbal	——	——	.52

Other correlations (.50 or more) involving these measures:
"Other" paraphasia $\times$ phrase length: .50

Within the speech-fluency cluster:
Phrase length $\times$ Articulation rating   .71
Other correlations of .50 or more:
Phrase Length $\times$ "Other" Paraphasia .50

Within the recitation-repetition cluster:

	Verbal Agility	Reciting	High-probability Repetition	Low-probability Repetition	Word Repetition
Automatized Sequence	.63	.26	.30	.39	.40
Verbal Agility	——	.35	.35	.34	.35
Reciting	——	——	.59	.52	.54
High-probability Repetition	——	——	——	.65	.61
Low-probability Repetition	——	——	——	——	.51

Other correlations involving these subtest scores:
High-probability Repetition $\times$ Spelled-word Recognition .53
Low-probability Repetition $\times$ Responsive Naming .52

Within the auditory-comprehension cluster:

	Body-part Identification	Commands	Complex Ideational Material
Word Discrimination	.61	.68	.62
Body-part Identification	——	.56	.55
Commands	——	——	.61

Other correlations involving subtests in this group:

Word Discrimination × Word-picture Matching	.59
Word Discrimination × Primer Dictation	.57
Word Discrimination × Word Recognition	.56
Body Parts × Primer-level Dictation	.62
Body Parts × Responsive Naming	.52
Body Parts × Comprehension of Oral Spelling	.50

It should be noted that three of the five above subtests outside the auditory-comprehension cluster, nevertheless depend on comprehension of auditory input (Word Recognition, Comprehension of Oral Spelling and Responsive Naming).

Within the word-finding cluster:

	Visual Confrontation Naming	Oral Word-reading	Animal-naming
Responsive Naming	.70	.49	.49
Visual Confrontation Naming	——	.74	.58
Oral Word-reading	——	——	.40

Other correlations with these subtests:

Responsive Naming × Body-part Comprehension	.52
Responsive Naming × Low-probability Repetition	.52
Visual Confrontation Naming × Oral Sentence-reading	.62
Visual Confrontation Naming × Primer-level Dictation	.54
Word-reading × Primer-level Dictation	.56

Within the reading cluster:

	Oral Sentences	Symbol-word Discrimination	Word Recognition	Comprehension of Oral Spelling	Word-picture Matching	Sentence and Paragraph Comprehension
Word-reading	.72	.52	.52	.48	.47	.54
Oral Sentences	——	.40	.38	.45	;38	.47
Symbol-word Discrimination	——	——	.60	.20	.63	.53
Phonetic Word Recognition	——	——	——	.39	.67	.60
Comprehension of Oral Spelling	——	——	——	——	.38	.45
Word-picture Matching	——	——	——	——	——	.66

Other correlations of subtests in this group:

Oral Sentence-reading × Confrontation Naming	.62
Symbol-word Discrimination × Word Discrimination	.52
Word Recognition × Serial Writing	.53
Word-picture Matching × Word Discrimination	.59
Word-picture Matching × Serial Writing	.53
Word-picture Matching × Primer-level Dictation	.58
Word-picture Matching × Written Confrontation Naming	.56
Comprehension of Oral Spelling × Primer-level Dictation	.61
Comprehension of Oral Spelling × Sentence to Dictation	.61
Comprehension of Oral Spelling × High-probability Repetition	.53
Comprehension of Oral Spelling × Body-part Identification	.50
Comprehension of Oral Spelling × Spelling to Dictation	.50

It is notable that of the nine different "nonreading" subtests listed here, five involve writing. Spelled-word comprehension has higher correlations within the writing cluster than the reading cluster.

Within the writing cluster:

	Spelling to Dictation	Written Confrontation Naming	Narrative Writing	Serial Writing	Primer-level Dictation	Sentence to Dictation
Writing Mechanics	.48	.48	.40	.55	.38	.40
Spelling to Dictation	—	.47	.54	.35	.56	.67
Written Confrontation Naming	—	—	.58	.38	.61	.59
Narrative Writing	—	—	—	.37	.40	.49
Serial Writing	—	—	—	—	.58	.38
Primer-level Dictation	—	—	—	—	—	.52

Other correlations involving these subtests:

Writing Mechanics × Word-picture Matching	.51
Written Confrontation Naming × Word-picture Matching	.56
Written Confrontation Naming × Oral Sentence-reading	.53
Serial Writing × Word-picture Matching	.53
Primer-level Dictation × Word Discrimination	.57
Primer-level Dictation × Body-part Identification	.62
Primer-level Dictation × Oral Sentence-reading	.59
Primer-level Dictation × Visual Confrontation Naming	.54
Primer-level Dictation × Comprehension of Oral Spelling	.61
Primer-level Dictation × Word-picture Matching	.58
Primer-level Dictation × Reading Sentence and Paragraph	.67
Sentence to Dictation × Comprehension of Oral Spelling	.61

It is noted that all these correlations with tasks outside the writing cluster are with reading tasks. The only exception is the case of Primer-level Dictation, which also correlates with auditory comprehension and naming tasks.

Within the spatial-quantitative cluster:

	Stick Memory	Total Finger	Right-left	Arithmetic	Clock	3-D Blocks
Drawing Comprehension	.48	.38	.31	.39	.35	.58
Stick Memory	—	.52	.50	.45	.58	.60
Total Finger	—	—	.47	.58	.51	.57
Right-left	—	—	—	.56	.57	.66
Arithmetic	—	—	—	—	.52	.59
Clock	—	—	—	—	—	.65

Other correlations involving these subtests:

Arithmetic × Word Recognition	.53
Arithmetic × Symbol and Word Discrimination	.53
Arithmetic × Word-picture Matching	.51
Arithmetic × Oral Sentence-reading	.55
Arithmetic × Written Confrontation Naming	.51
Arithmetic × Serial Writing	.52
Clock × Word Discrimination	.55
Clock × Commands	.60

FIRST FACTOR ANALYSIS (October 1966)

The scores were factor analyzed and subjected to orthogonal varimax rotation. Five factors emerged from this analysis. Subtests with loadings of .40 or more for each factor are listed in Table 3.

A large number of subtests loading on Factor I shows factor loadings of more than .50. These encompass the naming, auditory comprehension, reading and writing clusters. One would be tempted to call this a severity or, following Schuell and Jenkins, a general language factor. There is one contrary note. In the unrotated (principal components) factor analysis, the phrase-length rating has a negative loading of $-.31$ and the articulation rating, a negative loading of $-.19$. These are reduced to $-.15$ and $-.03$, respectively, after varimax rotation, although the makeup of the factor is not otherwise significantly affected in the rotation. This suggests that the configuration of Broca's aphasia is confounded with a severity factor to make up Factor I. This is probable because the principal features of Broca's aphasia are the relative preservation of the elementary naming, comprehension and reading responses in the context of a breakdown of articulation and fluency. Writing, like fluency, is usually impaired in Broca's aphasia and, in this respect, the high Factor I loadings of the writing tasks depart from that syndrome and are more readily accounted for by the severity of aphasia.

Factor II gives strong support to the concept of the clustering of spatial-quantitative-somatognosic tasks which are commonly associated with the intactness of the angular gyrus region of the left hemisphere.

Factor III represents the configuration of good articulation, fluency and all forms of paraphasia, along with impaired comprehension and repetition. This, as mentioned earlier, corresponds precisely to the components of Wernicke's aphasia and is an example of a factor whose emergence depends on the representation of sufficient patients of this type to permit the underlying positive and negative correlations to assert themselves.

Factor IV links fluency, ease of articulation and oral repetition of words and sentences. This group of functions represents the intactness of the elementary speech apparatus, as distinct from the processes which link speech to meaning. There is, in fact, a form of aphasia in which this system and this set of performances are well preserved—classical "transcortical sensory aphasia," called by Geschwind "isolation of the speech area." (For description of the syndrome, see Chapter 7.) While the syndrome is not often encountered in pure form, it is reasonable that its elements should be correlated.

Factor V has strong negative loadings, primarily on the subsections of the finger agnosia test, and links it with deficiencies in reading, writing, naming, right-left discrimination and arithmetic. It appears to represent the association, by anatomical contiguity, between the written language deficiencies of angular gyrus lesions and the elements of Gerstmann's syndrome (agraphia, right-left confusion, finger agnosia and acalculia). Anomia, being another neighborhood sign of the angular gyrus symptoms, appears in the form of poor confrontation naming.

Correlations vs. Factor Analysis

It is interesting to compare these two methods of establishing the associations among the subtests. The subtests of the paraphasia cluster include only two of six correlations of more than .50; the others all fall below .40. However, all members of this cluster are clearly marked by Factor III, where they appear in positive association with the two subtests of the fluency cluster and in negative association with the auditory comprehension and repetition clusters.

The fluency cluster appears in two factors—Factor III, where it has opposite loadings to those of the repetition scores and in Factor IV, where fluency, recitation and repetition

Table 3. Rotated Loadings of .40 or More for All Test Variables on Five Factors
(October 1966)

.40+ Rotated Factor I

Variable	Loading
Word Discrimination	.63
Body-part Identification	.51
Commands	.50
Complex Ideational Material	.43
Automatized Sequence	.46
Oral Sentence-reading	.54
High-probability Repetition	.41
Response Naming	.51
Visual Confrontation Naming	.64
Word-reading	.61
Symbol and Word Discrimination	.61
Comprehension of Oral Spelling	.67
Word-picture matching	.67
Sentence and Paragraph Reading	.61
Writing Mechanics	.59
Spelling to Dictation	.63
Written Confrontation Naming	.66
Narrative Writing	.59
Serial Writing	.59
Primer-level Dictation	.73
Sentences to Dictation	.62
Severity of Broca's component	

.40+ Rotated Factor II

Variable	Loading
Drawing to Comprehension	.68
Stick Memory	.62
Finger Comprehension	.41
Visual Finger-matching	.42
Total Fingers	.47
Right-left	.55
Arithmetic	.58
Clock-setting	.68
3-D Blocks	.81
Parietal Lobe Factor	

.40+ Rotated Factor III

Variable	Loading
Articulation Rating	.41
Phrase-length Rating	.50
Neologistic Paraphasia	.45
Literal Paraphasia	.40
Verbal Paraphasia	.54
"Other" Paraphasia	.64
Body-part Identification	-.45
Commands	-.42
Reciting	-.48
Low-probability Repetition	-.51
Responsive Naming	-.52
Animal-naming	-.40
Wernicke Factor	

.40+ Rotated Factor IV

Variable	Loading
Articulation Rating	.60
Phrase-length Rating	.44
Verbal Agility	.61
Automatized Sequence	.53
Word Repetition	.41
High-probability Repetition	.45
Low-probability Repetition	.42
Agility-repetition fluency	

.40+ Rotated Factor V

Variable	Loading
Oral Sentence-reading	-.47
Word-reading	-.45
Finger Comprehension	-.73
Finger-naming	-.61
Visual Finger-matching	-.40
Total Fingers	-.68

Table 4. Rotated Loadings of .40 or More for All Test Variables on Five Factors (October 1969)

Rotated Factor I (.40+) — Reading and Writing

Variable	Loading
Word-reading	.61
Visual Confrontation Naming	.57
Animal-naming	.41
Oral Sentence-reading	.72
Symbol and Word Discrimination	.47
Word Recognition	.47
Comprehension of Oral Spelling	.47
Word-picture Matching	.61
Sentence and Paragraph Reading	.75
Writing Mechanics	.59
Serial Writing	.67
Primer-level Dictation	.76
Spelling to Dictation	.81
Written Confrontation Naming	.72
Narrative Writing	.71
Sentence to Dictation	.71

Rotated Factor II (.40+) — Parietal Lobe

Variable	Loading
Draw to Comprehension	.76
Stick Memory	.69
Finger Comprehension	.56
Finger-naming	.51
Visual Finger-matching	.72
Tactile Finger Identification	.63
Total Fingers	.74
Right-left	.47
Arithmetic	.60
Clock-setting	.70
3-D Blocks	.76

Rotated Factor III (.40+) — Fluent-repetition Recitation

Variable	Loading
Articulation Rating	.65
Phrase-length Rating	.60
Verbal Agility	.78
Automatized Sequence Reciting	.71
Reciting	.58
Word Repetition	.66
High-probability Repetition	.76
Low-probability Repetition	.65
Responsive Naming	.61
Visual Confrontation Naming	.54

Rotated Factor IV (.40+) — Auditory Comprehension

Variable	Loading
Word Discrimination	-.78
Body-part Identification	-.79
Commands	-.74
Complex Ideational Material	-.71
Responsive Naming	-.55
Visual Confrontation Naming	-.43
Symbol and Word Discrimination	-.58
Word Recognition	-.62
Word-picture Matching	-.56
Sentence and Paragraph Reading	-.42
Serial Writing	-.51

Rotated Factor V (.40+) — Paraphasia

Variable	Loading
Literal Paraphasia	.55
Verbal Paraphasia	.71
"Other" Paraphasia	.57

are closely associated. If we were to regard factor loadings as purely an expression of common psychological properties, this would appear paradoxical. However, when we examine the way in which the aphasic syndromes produce alternative patterns of associations among subtests, the paradox disappears. In this case, we can regard Factor IV as the expression of a naturally associated system of skills, which is associated by the effect of Wernicke's aphasia. This disrupts the recognition of auditory input, interfering with repetition, but not affecting the mechanics of speech output as such. Thus, we are compelled to regard the results of our factor analysis as produced by an interaction of symptom clusters based on organic considerations and natural groupings based on psychological association.

The auditory comprehension cluster, which is clearly delineated in the intercorrelation matrix, does not appear as an independent factor. Rather it appears as a negatively loaded group in Factor III, which we consider the "Wernicke's aphasia" factor.

The word finding cluster is not clearly demarcated, either by the intercorrelation matrix or by the factor analysis. In the former, three of its subtests have correlations of more than .50 with auditory comprehension, repetition and writing. In the factor analysis, word finding ability appears primarily as a component of the overall severity of aphasia. Thus, the syndrome of anomic aphasia is not reflected in the factorial structure, presumably because there were not enough clear instances of this condition to affect the intercorrelations.

The reading and writing clusters show almost as much association as within each of the clusters in the intercorrelation matrix. However, the factor analysis picks them out as a group only insofar as they may be deficient in association with finger agnosia, right-left discrimination and arithmetic. Clinically, it is true, one rarely sees dramatic sparing of written language in a context of aphasia for spoken language. However, the syndrome of alexia and agraphia with min-

imal speech disturbance is well known and, as reflected in Factor V, is associated with other nonlinguistic symptoms of parietal lobe damage.

The cluster, spatial-constructional-quantitative-somesthetic-abilities, appears well defined both in the intercorrelation matrix and in Factor II—the most sharply defined of the factors. These are the subscores of the supplementary nonverbal battery, which we refer to as the "parietal lobe" battery. The cohesiveness of these scores, as opposed to their much weaker relationship to the language subtests, tends to vindicate the view that, taken as a group, they constitute evidence of a lesion in a discrete area of the brain.

SECOND FACTOR ANALYSIS
(October 1969)

In this larger sample of 189 aphasics based on precisely the same test procedures, we obtain a slightly different factorial structure from that of the earlier factor analysis. Table 4 lists under each factor the measures with loadings of .40 or more. Again, there are five interpretable factors, whose significance is more sharply defined than in the first analysis.

Factor I is related to scores on all the reading and writing subtests. Visual confrontation naming is the only measure outside of written language with a loading of more than .50 on this factor.

Factor II is related to performance on all the spatial-quantitative-somatognosic tests and minimally dependent on language tests proper; the only language performances with loadings of more than .30 are three simple writing measures. The diversity of impaired skills clustering in this factor (finger identification, calculation, clock-setting, block design) testifies to the validity of the belief that they are all mutually reinforcing indicators of a common site of brain lesion.

Factor III is determined by scores in verbal agility, fluency, repetition and recitation. Visual confrontation naming and responsive naming also have high loadings here (.54 and .61), as does severity (.64). This factor appears to represent the integrity of the mechanical automatisms of speech, and is inevitably associated with a mildness-severity dimension.

Factor IV is determined primarily by auditory comprehension scores, all with loadings of over .70. A secondary group of loadings of over .50 is associated with the reading scores. Responsive naming has a loading of .54. Thus, we may consider this to be an auditory comprehension factor or perhaps, more broadly, a receptive language factor.

Factor V is a clearly defined paraphasia factor which is based on three of the four paraphasia scores—literal paraphasia (.55), verbal paraphasia (.71) and "other" paraphasia (.57). The fourth paraphasia measure (neologistic) has a factor loading of .35. No other positive loadings reach .30, but the two sentence repetition measures have negative loadings of —.41 and —.32.

COMPARISON OF THE TWO FACTOR ANALYSES

The factors which emerge from the second analysis correspond more closely to the clusters of the intercorrelation matrix. Severity, which was the first factor in the first analysis, appeared as the major first factor only in the principal components factor analysis of the second analysis. After varimax rotation, the five factors correspond to relatively specific aspects of aphasic performance. The following comparisons may be noted between the first and second factor analyses.

1. Reading and writing, which were not isolated at all by the first analysis, now appear as a sharply defined first factor.

2. The "parietal lobe" or spatial-quantitative-somatognosic group remains as a clear Factor II.

3. Articulatory and grammatical fluency, which appeared as Factor IV on the first analysis, are represented as Factor III on the second.

4. Auditory comprehension and paraphasia, which appeared on a single "Wernicke's aphasia" factor (III) on the first analysis, are now clearly split into Factors IV and V, respectively.

The factors suggested by our test data correspond, in general, to clinical inferences about aphasia. That is, we have hitherto regarded written language as not entirely predictable from the level of spoken language, and have regarded fluency, auditory comprehension and paraphasia as interrelated, but capable of independent variation. Certainly, the diverse "parietal lobe functions" so clearly set apart in Factor II, have been regarded as a group of functions all pointing to a common cerebral locus.

These factors do not identify all the capacities whose isolated disturbance is occasionally noted. However, they appear to be sufficient to separate all the major aphasic syndromes, were they to be plotted in terms of the patients' factor scores. This is due largely to the fact that we have devised adequate measures of fluency and paraphasia. One glaring omission is the inability of the factor analysis to single out word-finding difficulty as an isolable feature, as it appears in "anomic aphasia." This is understandable, since all our scored measures of word production are a function of aphasia severity, regardless of type, and do not reflect the selective impairment of naming ability in the context of fluent output. Such a measure is derived from our rating-scale evaluation of word-finding, although these ratings were not included in the factor analysis.

The combination of articulatory facility, repetition and recitation in Factor III corresponds to the association of these functions clinically, but fails to reveal that there are instances in which they, too, vary independently. This is, of course, a basic limitation of the factor analytic technique, which is not responsive to the independent variation that occurs only in a few individuals.

Chapter 4

TEST PROCEDURES AND RATIONALE: MANUAL FOR THE BOSTON DIAGNOSTIC APHASIA TEST

This chapter constitutes an administrative manual, supplementing the instructions in the test booklet, where the latter are not self-explanatory.

Prior to administration of the test the vital background data necessary to orient the clinician to the educational, vocational and medical history of the patient should be recorded on the face sheet of the test booklet.

CONVERSATIONAL AND EXPOSITORY SPEECH

This section of the test booklet is designed to determine the level and quality of the patient's speech and comprehension under conditions of open-ended conversation and free narrative. If possible, it should be tape-recorded. Playback of the tape will greatly facilitate completing the Rating Scale Profile of Speech Characteristics. This scale covers those features which are most elusive to quantification, and will supplement the objective scores obtained from the rest of the examination.

Items "a" through "g" provide an inventory of common expressions available as responses in conversational give-and-take. They include the ability to reply appropriately to a greeting, to answer with "yes" or "no," to say "I think so," "I don't know," "I hope so" or their equivalents. The questions in the test booklet, suggested to elicit these expressions, need not be followed verbatim, particularly if the patient's level of speech is obviously above that demanded to answer them. Items "f" and "g" ask for

name and address and should always be included, since severely anomic patients may fail with these specific information-giving items in spite of being deceptively fluent in the opening small talk.

Item "h" places more demand on the patient for talking freely without a specific stimulus. Avoid asking "yes-no" questions in encouraging patient to elaborate, since these merely put a damper on conversation. Whenever possible, conversation should be continued about ten minutes. A sample of this length is likely to give the patient an opportunity to demonstrate his speech fluency, even though his opening conversation may be rather halting. However, many milder anomic patients begin to falter and make errors in speech after a beginning in which no speech difficulty is apparent for several minutes. The degree of fluency should be judged in terms of the subject's best performance.

The conversation is terminated at the discretion of the examiner, who then presents item "i"—a picture situation (the Cookie Theft) with instructions to "Tell all about what you see going on in this picture." If a tape recording is being made to facilitate rating, it should be continued through the picture description. It will be noted that the quality of the speech pattern often changes drastically in the shift from free conversation to picture description. The reason is that some anomic patients have the knack of moving about from one available expression to another in free conversation, while completely avoiding the words that they sense as a source of trouble. The vocabulary constraints of the picture bring out the word-finding difficulty more sharply.

Use of Rating Scale Profile, Severity Rating and Z-score Profile

Six features of speech production, which are not satisfactorily measured by objective scores, are to be rated during, or immediately after, concluding the conversational and expository speech interview. If a tape recording has been made, rating may be deferred and done during a playback of the recording, which is preferable to rating the live interview. Rating is done more reliably when the rater can concentrate on listening for the critical features which may escape him when he is busy interviewing.

The six features are: melodic line, phrase length, articulatory agility, grammatical form (variety of grammatical constructions), paraphasia in running speech and word-finding. In addition, a seventh scale of auditory comprehension is based on a conversion of the objective test scores. Five of the ratings are on a seven point scale on which "7" stands for minimum abnormality and "1" stands for maximum abnormality. The scale for word-finding ability is deviant at both extremes, as explained below.

The severity rating is a scale of capacity for oral communication ranging from "0" for "no communication possible" to "5" for "no perceptible handicap." The Profile of Speech Characteristics must be interpreted in the light of the severity rating. The steps of the severity rating are defined on the scale record form (Figure 2).

The z-score profile, also included in the test booklet, provides a summary of the raw scores for each subtest of the Boston Diagnostic Aphasia Test, as well as the ratings assigned for severity, articulation and phrase length. The position of the raw score on its horizontal line may be read off as a z-score from the scale at the top and bottom of the page. The z-score gives the deviation

above or below the mean $(z=0)$, in standard deviation units. This permits a direct comparison of performance level on tests whose raw scores may have totally disparate ranges.

How to Assign Profile Ratings

MELODIC LINE. This term refers to the intonational pattern, which normally encompasses the entire sentence. In the most severely dysrhythmic speech there may be no intonational link, even between syllables; words are spoken as though being enumerated, rather than grouped syntactically. At the intermediate level (4), normal melodic line may extend to three- or four-word expressions of a stereotyped nature, such as, "I don't know" or "I can't say it." Patients whose sentences never exceed four words in length can only obtain a rating of (4) as maximum. Two interpolated steps are provided between the midpoint and each extreme.

PHRASE LENGTH. This quality is measured by the length of uninterrupted runs of words, set off at either end by a pause or sentence boundary. The numerical steps of the scale represent the longest number of words per run which occurs at least once in about ten starts by the patient. Thus, this rating is *not* the average length of uninterrupted word groupings, but the longest grouping which may be expected occasionally. If, for example, in thirty utterances, three contain six or more words without a break, the scale rating is "6," even if one of the occasions extended to ten words and even though the majority of the utterances are aborted after three to four words. The criterion of one in ten is given as a guide for estimation by the rater. For the degree of precision expected in this rating, it is not necessary to count utterances.

VERBAL AGILITY. The ease with which the patient articulates phonemic sequences constitutes verbal agility. The examiner should listen for any awkwardness, explosive attack, groping in initial sounds, simplification of consonant blends or sound substitutions *due to articulatory difficulty*. If every word is

Patient's Name _____ Date of rating _____

Rated by _____

APHASIA SEVERITY RATING SCALE

0. No usable speech or auditory comprehension.

1. All communication is through fragmentary expression; great need for inference, questioning and guessing by the listener. The range of information which can be exchanged is limited, and the listener carries the burden of communication.

2. Conversation about familiar subjects is possible with help from the listener. There are frequent failures to convey the idea, but patient shares the burden of communication with the examiner.

3. The patient can discuss <u>almost all everyday problems</u> with little or no assistance. However, reduction of speech and/or comprehension make conversation about certain material difficult or impossible.

4. Some obvious loss of fluency in speech or facility of comprehension, without significant limitation on ideas expressed or form of expression.

5. Minimal discernible speech handicaps; patient may have subjective difficulties which are not apparent to listener.

RATING SCALE PROFILE OF SPEECH CHARACTERISTICS

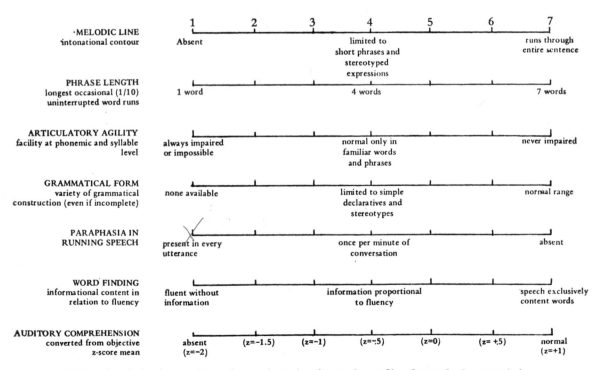

FIGURE 2.   Aphasia severity rating scale and rating scale profile of speech characteristics.

26

produced with normal ease, the patient receives a maximum score here. Literal paraphasia, i.e., sound transpositions or contaminations in a setting of facile articulation, does not constitute a loss of verbal agility for purposes of this rating. The rating is based on the prevalence, as much as the severity, of impaired articulation. A rating of "1" indicates articulatory difficulty in every utterance. The middle score of "4" indicates that articulation is normal only in brief, relatively overlearned expressions. Two interpolated steps are provided between the midpoint and each extreme.

GRAMMATICAL FORM. This encompasses the continuum from "agrammatic" or one-word sentence speech to a normal variety of grammatical forms. At severe levels, isolated nouns predominate and one rarely hears syntactic combinations beyond verb plus object. The verb is usually unmarked with respect to tense. At moderate levels, the patient constructs simple declarative sentences in the present or past tense, but does not deviate from the "subject-verb-object" sequence and never starts a sentence with a subordinate clause. At normal levels, one hears longer sentences with subordinate clauses, conditionals, future tenses and passive constructions. Many patients who use a variety of grammatical forms may leave sentences incomplete because of word-finding difficulty; in addition, their grammar may be flawed by their semantic misusage of words (paraphasia). Paraphasic errors and aborted sentences are compatible with normal ratings for "variety of grammatical construction."

PARAPHASIA IN RUNNING SPEECH. The focus here is not on paraphasic substitutions of individual nouns in one-word responses as seen in aphasics of many types, but rather on the substitutions or insertions of semantically erroneous words in running conversation, which is diagnostically significant. For this scale, not only semantic errors but partially or completely neologistic errors are noted, and the score depends chiefly on the prevalence of such errors. The maximum abnormality of "1" implies paraphasia included in every utterance; the minimum of "7" implies complete absence of such errors. This score "7" is also assigned to patients who have no runs of fluent speech. The midpoint of "4" represents an average of a paraphasic error in each minute of conversation.

WORD-FINDING. The patient's capacity to evoke needed concept names is reflected in the informational content of his speech; however, the rating is made with respect to the level of fluency. In a quantitative sense, it reflects the proportion of substantives and specific action-words to the number of low-information words, i.e., grammatical connectives, pronouns, auxiliary verbs, indefinite words such as "something" and other compounds of "thing," "place," "body." A rating of "7" stands for speech consisting almost exclusively of substantives and picturable actions. The relative dearth of low-information words is usually reflected in short or agrammatic sentence forms, a characteristic which tends to correlate with this scale. The middle rating of "4" means that the examiner estimates the proportion of specific nouns and verbs to be just appropriate to the fluency level. A rating of "1" indicates fluent speech in which virtually no specific nouns or verbs occur. Such speech, which we call "empty speech," is usually grammatically organized, but vague and circumlocutory, with the same expressions recurring frequently.

Unlike the other scales, this one does not represent normal performance at step "7" and most deviant at step "1." In fact, the patient rated "7" may have great difficulty in naming. The rating of "7" indicates only that the naming function is so much better preserved than grammatical fluency that his output consists almost entirely of content-words.

AUDITORY COMPREHENSION. Unlike the other variables on this profile chart, this can be adequately measured by objective test

scores. Nevertheless, it was included on
the chart because of its contribution to the
distinctive appearance of profiles of the
various diagnostic groups of aphasics. The
entry on this scale is based on the mean
score of the four auditory comprehension
subtests, as plotted on the z-score summary
profile. Since the possible range of mean
z-scores for auditory comprehension is from
−2 to +1, the following conversion table
(reproduced on the rating scale) is provided:

Scale	1	2	3	4	5	6	7
Z-score	−2	−1.5	−1	−.5	0	+.5	+1

Reliability of the Ratings

In the development of the Profile of Speech
Characteristics, judgments were made independently by three raters, listening to the
tape-recorded conversation. The ratings
used were the mean of the three judges'
ratings for each scale. In order to assess
the reliability of the individual judges' ratings,
we computed Pearson product moment correlations, across ninety-nine subjects, between the two most disparate ratings on each
scale, this being the most stringent approach
possible. The correlation coefficients were
as follows:

Melodic Line	.85
Phrase Length	.90
Articulatory Agility	.90
Grammatical Form	.90
Paraphasia in Running Speech	.79
Word finding	.78

The last (auditory comprehension) scale
is based on the mean of the four auditory
subtest scores which have reliability coefficients of .96, .68, .91 and .89, thus assuring
an adequate reliability for this scale.

The relatively low reliability of the word-
finding and paraphasia ratings corresponds
to the subjective uncertainty of the judges in
making these ratings. However, in view of
the method of obtaining the reliability
coefficients, it is felt that they are minimal
estimates and that we are on safe ground in
having the individual examiner make each
rating.

AUDITORY COMPREHENSION

Word Discrimination

This is a multiple-choice, auditory word-
recognition test. It samples six semantic
categories of words: objects, geometric
forms, letters, actions, numbers and colors,
giving the opportunity to observe selective
impairment of word categories. This test
correlates best with the other three auditory
comprehension scores (.71 with Body-part
Identification, .68 with Commands and .62
with Complex Ideational Material).

ADMINISTRATION AND SCORING. Each of
the two test cards presents three categories
of visual stimuli and the examiner names
words in rotation among these three categories, forcing the subject to shift his cate-
gory-set with each test word. Card 2
(Objects, Forms, Letters) is presented first,
then Card 3 (Actions, Numbers, Colors).
The stimulus question is always in the form,
"Show me_____." Scoring allows full
credit of two points for correct identification
within five seconds, partial credit of one
point for correct identification after more
than five seconds (self-correction is permitted), partial credit of half a point for
location of the correct category (Column
"Cat." on record sheet). If the patient does
not locate the correct category, he is directed
to it on the card and, if he then succeeds, is
allowed partial credit of half a point (under
Column "Cue"). One half point for "Cat."
is allowed whether the subject points to the
wrong member of the correct category or
merely points in the correct group without
making a choice. Examiner should record
all incorrect choices in writing. Maximum
score possible is seventy-two.

Body-part Identification

Because of the frequent selective disturbance of body-part comprehension, a larger,
separate sampling of this group of words is
included. The first eighteen items sample a
wide range of difficulty in body-part names,
including three fingers (middle, index and

thumb). Eight items are included for right-left comprehension. This subtest's highest three intercorrelations are within the auditory comprehension cluster: .71 with Word Discrimination, .68 with Commands and .62 with Complex Ideational Material.

ADMINISTRATION AND SCORING. The patient is asked to point on his own body to the part named by the examiner, with the command, "Show me your_____." While finger identification and right-left discrimination are not scored separately, they deserve special attention as a screening test for disorders of parietal lobe function, in which these concepts may be selectively disturbed. (A more exhaustive test of finger identification and right-left discrimination is included in a supplement to this manual as part of a battery for parietal lobe functions.)

Full credit of one point is allowed for each of the first eighteen items, if identified within five seconds; one-half point is allowed for response of over five seconds' latency. Up to two additional points are earned for right-left comprehension, for a total possible raw score of twenty. In scoring right-left discrimination, only the side of the body is relevant. Patient may point to his right eye instead of "right cheek" without loss of credit.

Commands

In this subtest, the capacity to process increasingly concentrated auditory information is tested with commands ranging from one significant informational unit to five. Carrying out commands and even pointing, as required in the preceding subtest, presuppose the preservation of the ability to carry out purposeful movements, i.e., the absence of severe *apraxia*. Since apraxia often accompanies aphasia, this possible source of contamination must be borne in mind, particularly if the patient does disproportionately well in the next subtest, which requires only the answering of "yes-no" questions. The highest intercorrelations of this subtest are also within the auditory

comprehension cluster: .68 with Word Discrimination, .61 with Complex Ideational Material and .58 with Body-part Identification.

ADMINISTRATION AND SCORING. Each command may be repeated once, on request; however, the command must be repeated as a whole. Each underlined element in each command in the test booklet may be passed or failed independently, permitting a score of zero to fifteen.

Complex Ideational Material

This subtest requires the patient to understand and express agreement or disagreement concerning factual material that does not relate to a stimulus immediately before him. Starting with simple facts ("Will a board sink in water?" "Will a stone sink in water?"), the material increases in length and in the demand for reference to knowledge or easy inferences beyond the mere recall of the words. Thus there is an intellectual component which, however, does not go beyond average adult ability, even at the most difficult level. The intercorrelations with other subtests are highest with the other three auditory comprehension subtests.

ADMINISTRATION AND SCORING. Each item consists of a pair of questions, one requiring "no" and the other, "yes." The order of "yes" and "no" questions is randomized. Both questions must be answered correctly for credit to be earned for the item. Items five through twelve are based on the comprehension of a series of four paragraphs, with two items (each consisting of a pair of "yes"-"no" questions) based on each paragraph, presented immediately after the paragraph is read.

One point is allowed for each item with both questions correctly answered, for a maximum of twelve.

ORAL EXPRESSION

This section begins with the testing of the mechanics of articulation and proceeds from a test of automatized "nonpropositional" speech, through repetition, to progressively more information-carrying acts of word-finding. While tests of sentence repetition and sentence reading are included, the formulation of connected speech is not tested here, but must be evaluated from the free conversation and narrative. The final subtest is a measure of word-production fluency in controlled association.

Nonverbal Agility

This subtest is aimed at providing a comparison between nonverbal use of the lips and tongue as opposed to articulation in actual speech. Contrary to widely held opinion, this correlation is not very great. The test consists of a set of six alternating movements, such as protruding and retracting the tongue repeatedly, or alternately pursing and releasing the lips. Poor performance here reflects incoordination and weakness of the speech musculature which contributes to the nonaphasic dysarthria which may complicate the symptom complex in some patients. Correlations with the remainder of the language subtests are all below .30.

ADMINISTRATION AND SCORING. Each movement is done after a verbal instruction and demonstration. Full credit of two points or half credit of one point depends on the number of full alternations done in five seconds, timed by the second hand of a watch.

Verbal Agility

Because of the facilitation afforded by repetition, single-word repetition tests are often quite well done by patients whose natural speech is dysarthric. On the other hand, they may be failed by "fluent" aphasics, who produce paraphasic distortions on repetition.

The approach of this subtest is to bypass both of these sources of error. First, by timing the rate of serial repetitions of the same word, defects which are inaudible in

a single-word repetition are reflected in the slowing of serial performance. Second, by aiding the patient to attain initial correct repetition, we overcome the spuriously low scores in articulation which are due to paraphasia. The one important intercorrelation with another subtest of the battery is .63 with Automatized Sequences.

ADMINISTRATION AND SCORING. Some patients may be aided in getting started by seeing the written word. Card 4 is provided for this purpose and the examiner points to each word as it is presented orally. When a patient is prevented by paraphasia or poor comprehension from correctly initiating his repetitions, the item is invalidated. Rejection of more than two items for this reason invalidates the score of this subtest.

Two points or one point per item are earned, depending on the number of correct repetitions of the test word within a five-second interval. If one or two items are invalidated, prorate the score on the basis of 7/5 or 7/6, as appropriate.

SCORING OF ARTICULATION AND PARAPHASIA. Seven of the following subtests provide for a tally of articulatory difficulty and paraphasic errors for each response. Paraphasia and articulatory difficulty (dysarthria) are mutually exclusive classifications. While there are "gray areas" in which a decision between them is difficult, the principle underlying the two concepts is important to master.

Articulatory difficulty refers to loss of accuracy in forming individual phonemes, so that the sounds which emerge—particularly difficult consonants and blends—are not standard English phonemes. This usually occurs in a context of effort, awkwardness and slowness of speech. Occasionally, one hears "infantilisms," such as "ts" for "ch" or "w" for "r." It is in relation to "literal paraphasia" that the confusion with dysarthria is most likely. In the case of literal paraphasia, individual phonemes and syllables are easily produced and are perceived by the listener as standard English phonemes, but their selection and ordering in a word is incorrect.

In scoring, responses which are correct in content receive a tally under the appropriate articulation column:

Normal

Stiff but correct: no transcribable phonemic error.

Distorted: at least one definite phonemic distortion, but word still recognizable.

Failure: not recognizable due to articulatory difficulty, but discernible as an attempt at the target word.

Paraphasic errors should be tallied even when self-corrected. The four columns on the right side of the page provide an opportunity to tally paraphasia under four headings. The first three columns on the right refer to paraphasic errors referable to known target words.

1. *Neologistic distortion*—Introduction of extraneous phonemes or transposition of intended phonemes so that less than half of the intended word is discernible as an intact unit. In the extreme, distortions may take the form of neologistic jargon.

2. *Literal paraphasia*—Transposition or introduction of extraneous phonemes such that more than half of the intended word is produced as an intact unit.

3. *Verbal paraphasia*—Substitution of an inappropriate word during the effort to say a particular target word. Perseveration of a previously used word is included here, but only once for any perseverated word.

4. *Other*—A number of types of paraphasia which involve extended speech sequences. It also is used for some types of nonparaphasic, inappropriate responses, defined below. The abbreviation of the category should be written into the column.

enj.—extended neologistic jargon: running speech including neologistic expressions

eej.—extended English jargon: running speech composed of English words in a meaningless sequence

irrel.—irrelevant speech which is not jargon, but inappropriate

cl.—circumlocution

The use of recurrent stereotyped syllables or words is not scored as paraphasia.

The total number of paraphasias checked under each column is totalled for the oral-expression subtests on Automatized Sequences through Body-part Naming and entered on the z-score summary chart. The pattern of the breakdown of paraphasias, particularly the relative incidence of literal paraphasia, contributes to the diagnostic classification. (See Chapter 7 for a discussion of syndromes and case illustrations.)

Automatized Sequences

In this subtest, four well overlearned sequences are tested: days of the week, months of the year, numbers from one to twenty-one and the alphabet. Recitation of memorized sequences is commonly better preserved than propositional speech, and this is usually true for aphasics of all types. Especially dramatic discrepancies in favor of recitation are found in transcortical aphasics. (See Chapter 7.) The only correlation of over .50 observed is one of .63 with Verbal Agility.

ADMINISTRATION AND SCORING. Many patients succeed only when the first word is supplied, and no credit is lost for help in initiating a series. The patient may be assisted by prompting in the middle of a series, but no more than four items should be supplied before discontinuing. The test booklet shows from three to nine words per line, and this *may* lead to multiple entries of articulation and paraphasia on each line. No more than one check should be entered in any column, but as many different columns as are needed may be checked to record the level of articulation and types of paraphasia produced with the words on a given line.

Two points maximum are allowed for complete recitation of any series and one point partial credit is allowed for unaided runs of consecutive words of various lengths as follows: days—four consecutive; months —five consecutive; numbers— eight consecutive; alphabet—seven consecutive; maximum score—8.

Recitation, Singing and Rhythm

The trio of performances sampled in this section were grouped together because of their apparent relationship to musical ability; however, intercorrelations between them are very low. Reciting "nursery rhymes" has correlation coefficients in the .50's with scores based on word and sentence repetition, but rhythm-tapping and melody are largely independent of language skills and of each other. While, clinically, the ability to sing a melody correctly is usually preserved in severe aphasics, the ability to produce the words with it is much less common and characterizes "transcortical" aphasics, in whom the remarkable preservation of verbal recitation is associated with selective sparing of repetition.

Thus, while the presumed common contribution of these three performances to musical ability is unproved, we have continued to group them in a single section, with three separate rating-scale scores.

ADMINISTRATION AND SCORING. *Recitation.* Several nursery rhymes are suggested to elicit completion responses. Occasionally, a patient takes offense at being presented with childish content, but this reaction can be avoided by explaining, "Many of our patients who have trouble talking find it easy to say things they learned when they were small. I am going to let you hear some nursery rhymes that you probably remember, and see if you can go on where I leave off." It is suggested that the Lord's Prayer be tried as an alternative, or in addition, to the nursery rhymes.

Melody. Since many adults are reticent about singing alone, the examiner should start the song, encouraging the patient by gesture to join, and then sing softly enough to hear how accurately the patient carries the melody. If the patient has a preferred song, he may sing that instead of "My country 'tis of thee" (America).

Tapping rhythms. Four rhythmic patterns are tapped with a pencil by the examiner for the patient to imitate. The first three are simple cyclic patterns which are tapped over and over through six cycles: first: ◡ ' ◡ ' second: ' ◡◡ ' ◡◡ third: ◡ '' ◡ ''. The fourth is the familiar rhythm of the jingle, "Shave and a haircut, two bits": ' ◡◡ '' , ''.

Recitation, melody and rhythm are each scored on a three-step rating scale from zero (fail), through one (impaired), to two (good).

Repetition of Words

Word repetition is an easy task, and only the most severely impaired patients fail it completely. Failure may be due to poor comprehension, as is frequently the case in Wernicke's aphasia and even more markedly so in the rare instances of word-deafness. The arousal of a fragment of the auditory image will be reflected in well-articulated, but paraphasic, responses in which a fragment of the word can be identified. Occasionally, the sound of the stimulus word appears to be lost immediately, while the patient has grasped and retained some of its meaning. His effort to repeat emerges as a verbal paraphasia, i.e., a word related by connotation to the stimulus.

Another source of failure to repeat is severe incapacitation of the motor speech output system, auditory word recognition being adequate. In such cases, speech output is reduced to little more than a few highly overlearned expressions, if that. Of course, loss of comprehension may coexist with impaired motor output. so that careful exploration is needed before ascribing a cause to failure of repetition.

Finally, repetition failure may occur with fluent spontaneous speech and normal auditory comprehension in *conduction aphasia.* In this disorder, literal paraphasia interferes with repetition, but rarely at the level of single common English words. The highest correlations of this subtest are with repetition of high-probability phrases (.61) and with recitation of nursery rhymes (.54).

ADMINISTRATION AND SCORING. In this subtest, a wide sampling of word types is presented, including a grammatical function word, objects, colors, a letter, numbers, an abstract verb of three syllables and a tongue twister (Methodist Episcopal). Notation of articulation and paraphasia is made in the appropriate column. An item is scored correct if all phonemes are in correct order and recognizable. One point is allowed per item for a total of ten.

Repeating Phrases and Sentences

This section is divided into two separately scored sets of sentences, differing in vocabulary difficulty and predictability of the verbal content, and referred to as "high-probability" and "low-probability" sentences. For example, at the five-word level, a high-probability sentence is, "You should not tell her"; a low-probability sentence is, "Pry the tin lid off." The separation of the test into two sets is based on previous findings which showed that patients with severe anomic aphasia have an enormous overdependence on the predictability of the content, with resulting discrepancies between high-probability and low-probability scores. Nevertheless, the correlation between the two scores is fairly high (.65). Since repetition of sentences is a complex operation depending on many components, the diagnostic significance of this subtest depends on its relation to other performances. When it is deviantly high in comparison with naming and comprehension, it is indicative of transcortical aphasia; when deviantly low in comparison with phrase length and comprehension, it is indicative of conduction aphasia.

ADMINISTRATION AND SCORING. The sentences must be read as an uninterrupted unit for patient to repeat, alternating between a high-probability and a low-probability item. For credit on any item, all words must be reproduced without paraphasic errors, but articulatory distortions consistent with the patient's general articulatory difficulty are not penalized.

One point is allowed for each sentence correctly repeated and high- and low-probability sections are scored separately from zero to eight.

Word-reading

This is a test of word-finding which is, however, dependent on basic reading ability. If subsequent testing shows that the patient no longer recognizes written language, this score must be interpreted purely in that light. However, it is possible for the written word to be understood and failed orally for two reasons. The meaning may be grasped or partially grasped without arousing an auditory component sufficient to guide the final speech output. In this case, the patient may respond with a word related in meaning to the stimulus, e.g., saying "green" for "brown" or "square" for "circle." Alternatively, he may associate phonetically to part of a word, with or without grasping its meaning, e.g., saying "char" for "chair." On the other hand, he may fully appreciate the phonetic structure of the stimulus, yet fail because of inability to mobilize the motor speech system, as in the case of the patient who can articulate few words under any conditions.

As a test of word-finding, word-reading is easier than confrontation naming for some patients because the written word directly arouses phonetic associations without the necessity for mediation by comprehension, or the intent to express the meaning of the word. Understandably, the .74 correlation with Visual Confrontation Naming is on a par with that for Oral Sentence-reading (.76).

ADMINISTRATION AND SCORING. The words are read from Card 5 as the examiner points in succession to each one. Full credit is allowed for response within three seconds and partial credit for response in three to ten seconds or ten to thirty seconds. The examiner checks under the column heading corresponding to the time delay. The examiner's estimate of the delay gives sufficient precision in scoring. The use of a stopwatch is unnecessarily cumbersome. Paraphasia and articulation are to be checked for each response. The maximum score of thirty is based on three points full credit on each item. Partial credits are added according to the response delay indicated in the column heading in which response is recorded.

Responsive Naming

In this approach to word-finding, an orally presented question serves as the stimulus. The response words include nouns (watch, scissors, match, drugstore), colors (green, black), verbs (shave, wash, write) and a number (twelve). While performance here obviously depends on a certain minimum of auditory comprehension, its closest correlation is with Visual Confrontation Naming (.70). This supports the concept of word-finding as a separate component of language, whether stimulus input is by spoken word or picture. When the z-score for performance on this test is much below that for Visual Confrontation Naming, it is usually due to impaired auditory comprehension.

It should be noted that the stimulus questions usually contain a key word which is a close associate of the expected response. For those patients who have exceptionally strong verbal-associative skills, performance in this task may exceed that for Visual Confrontation Naming.

ADMINISTRATION AND SCORING. As in the other naming subtests, the score depends on the time interval required to produce the response, and a check is entered for any correct response, under the column heading (0–3″, 3–10″, 10–30″) corresponding to the approximate response delay, as estimated by the examiner. In case of a paraphasic response, the record should show what was said and a tally check entered in the appropriate paraphasia column. For correct responses, the quality of articulation should be entered. Total the number of points (3, 2, 1 or 0) corresponding to the columns which are checked. Maximum score possible is thirty.

Visual Confrontation Naming

Naming to visual presentation is a universally used test for aphasia since virtually all aphasic patients have some loss of capacity to perform. While it may be described as a visual input-oral output task, there is reason to believe that this is a simplistic view which does not do justice to the intervening processes. The form taken by the errors gives some inkling as to where and how the naming process is going astray. Thus, patients whose difficulty is primarily at the speech-output stage are likely to show difficulties in articulation which are relieved by having the word supplied by the examiner. They are self-critical and discriminate sharply between the correct and erroneous response. Those who fail to evoke the correct inner auditory pattern are more likely to produce paraphasic mistakes. When the correct word is offered them, it may not register as correct, even though their auditory comprehension is excellent in other contexts. Thus, there is evidence in some patients of a two-way dissociation between the concept and the word. Patients whose paraphasia is confined to phonemic substitutions and transpositions are usually acutely aware of their errors, but have the same difficulty when offered the word for repetition. These are the "conduction aphasics," discussed in a later chapter.

The stimulus items on Cards 2 and 3 are the same ones used in the word-discrimination test, and include objects, geometric forms, letters, actions, numbers, colors and body parts. These various categories are often unevenly affected by aphasia. Letter- and number-naming are most often spared, while object-naming is least often spared

(Goodglass, Klein, Carey and Jones, 1966). While, for quantitative purposes, the total score is the only measure of achievement on this test, the examiner should attend to the above-mentioned qualitative features, i.e., relationship among the word categories, category of paraphasia, if any, and response to assistance in saying intended words.

ADMINISTRATION AND SCORING. The examiner estimates the reaction time for each correct response and enters a check in the column labeled with the corresponding time interval. The maximum score obtainable for the 35 items is 105. Paraphasias should be tallied and entered verbatim for later reference. Articulation level should be tallied for all correct responses.

Body-part Naming

This addition to the confrontation-naming subtest, expanding the examination of body-part naming, was devised to determine whether the common selective impairment of body-part comprehension has its counterpart in the naming sphere. This subsection is in experimental form and no information on its intercorrelations is yet available.

ADMINISTRATION AND SCORING. The examiner points to the body part to be named *on himself*, and scores as in the preceding section. Maximum score is thirty.

Animal-naming (Fluency in Controlled Association)

A further approach to word-finding is that of measuring fluency in controlled association. This is a widely used technique in clinical testing and it appears in two forms in the Stanford-Binet: once in the form of unrestricted word-naming and once in the form of animal-naming. The procedure suggested here is an adaptation of the Stanford-Binet procedure for animal-naming, modified by giving the subject preliminary instructions to consider animals of all varieties and finally giving a starting word, "dog." The purpose of these instructions is to facilitate the task in two ways: first, to provide a

preliminary set which may assist the subject in shifting from one category to another and, second, to provide a definite starting point for timing, since many aphasics have inordinate difficulty in initiating a chain of associations, yet have reasonable fluency once under way.

The norm for ten-year-old children is twelve different animals in sixty seconds. Average adults name about eighteen. Performance in this type of test is reduced not only in aphasics, but in many brain-injured patients whose rate of ideation and ability to shift are impaired. While most normals start off naming rapidly in the first fifteen seconds, then taper off, aphasics more frequently run out of associations early and recover repeatedly with another burst of words.

This subtest has its highest correlation (.58) with Visual Confrontation Naming, dropping to a .49 correlation with Responsive Naming. It has a high negative correlation (−.44) with the phrase-length rating because, when severity is controlled, aphasics with the highest fluency in connected speech are the most deficient in word-finding.

ADMINISTRATION AND SCORING. The instructions to the patient are given in the wording provided in the test booklet and the examiner starts timing when he provides "dog" as the first word. Words are listed under the fifteen-second grouping columns provided in the test booklet and ninety seconds are allowed for naming. The score consists of the number of different words named in the most productive consecutive sixty-second period.

Oral Sentence-reading

Reading connected material aloud goes beyond the requirements for reading detached words in that it places a demand on the patient's command of grammatical forms. The small grammatical words and inflectional endings are often omitted by those patients who omit them in spontaneous speech. This complex task is included, not so much because of its value as an analytic technique, but because the interaction of many component factors makes this performance difficult to predict unless it is tested directly. For example, a high degree of accomplishment in phonetic association may overcome a severe aphasia and result in surprisingly good performance. The word-reading test is subject to the same underlying skill and, naturally enough, these tests correlate strongly (.76).

ADMINISTRATION AND SCORING. Sentences are read from Cards 6 and 7. A sentence-reading task offers great temptation to allow part credit for nearly correct performance. Because this would raise as many scoring problems as it would solve, a simple all-or-none score was decided on for each sentence. No credit is lost for articulatory awkwardness which is consistent with the patient's speech, but no transpositions of sounds or other paraphasic intrusions are permitted. Score zero to ten, one point per sentence.

UNDERSTANDING WRITTEN LANGUAGE

The subtests of this section focus on a number of the elementary associative skills which either underlie reading or are by-products of the way we learn to read. For example, recognition of the equivalence of letters written in various styles is a necessary and universal accomplishment of the normal reader, while recognition of oral spelling is a by-product, not a part, of the normal reading process, yet one which is a sign of the intactness of the reading apparatus. Comprehension of connected material is tested by an untimed multiple-choice test. There is no attempt to measure speed and efficiency at the upper levels of reading skill, where a speed test would encroach on the range of normal adult reading ability.

Symbol and Word Discrimination

A prerequisite to reading comprehension is the recognition of letters as familiar symbols, apart from recalling their names or phonetic value. Our means of testing this

function is the multiple-choice matching of letters and short words across different styles of writing—upper- and lower-case cursive, and printed. This is a purely visual recognition task, yet its intimate relationship with the mechanics of reading is demonstrated by the fact that its highest correlation (.61) is with the task of matching spoken to written words. The next four highest correlations are within the group of reading subtests. In difficulty, it is on a low level, and missing more than one item usually corresponds to severe reading difficulty.

ADMINISTRATION AND SCORING. The two Cards, 8 and 9, contain the ten items. In each case, the examiner points to the model word or letter centered above the five multiple-choice responses and asks the subject to select the equivalent. If the patient's auditory comprehension is defective, he may usually be led to understand by pantomime, using the first item as a demonstration. Scoring is one point per item, zero to ten.

Phonetic Association

The link between sound and letter is tested by two procedures separately scored, Word Recognition and Comprehension of Oral Spelling.

WORD RECOGNITION. This subtest was designed to reveal the intactness of auditory-visual phonetic associations without necessarily involving either comprehension or verbalization by the patient. The task is to select, from a multiple choice of five written words, the one spoken by the examiner. A second feature is built into this task which occasionally reveals a striking phenomenon—the ability to respond to the connotative meaning of a written word *without* appreciating its phonetic value. Examination of the multiple-choice sets shows that in four items the incorrect choices consist of three words connotatively similar to the test word and only one word similar in structure. Thus, for the second item, "pond," the four incorrect words are "lake," "water," "creek" and "fond." In the remaining four items, the proportion is reversed, i.e., three words are structurally similar and one is related by meaning. For example, for the first item, "ship," the four incorrect choices are "shop," "slip," "skip" and "boat." While the ability to associate between a concept and a written word without an inner phonetic experience is occasionally found at the one-word level, we have discussed earlier the evidence that normal reading does involve phonetic mediation. The intercorrelations of this subtest are primarily within the reading cluster, with the highest correlation of .67 with Word-picture Matching.

Administration and scoring. Using Cards 10 and 11, the examiner instructs the patient to find the one word, out of five on a line, which matches the word the examiner says. The words are given in the order they appear in the test booklet. Score one point for each correct answer for a maximum of eight.

COMPREHENSION OF ORAL SPELLING. Understanding orally spelled words is obviously not a part of the normal reading process. We might entirely question its relevance in aphasia were it not that (1) it is universally acquired in the usual course of acquisition of written language and (2) it is a very fragile skill in the face of some cases of aphasia, even with patients who read adequately on written presentation. While this task demands the participation of auditory comprehension, its highest correlations (both .61) are with the ability to write simple words from dictation and the ability to write sentences from dictation.

Administration and scoring. The patient is asked to listen while a word is spelled aloud to him and then immediately to say or otherwise indicate what it is. The words should be spelled at about two letters per second. If the patient appears to recognize a word but cannot express it, it may be offered as a multiple choice, with several similar-sounding words, for him to identify. The multiple-choice procedure is open to guesswork, for it may permit the patient to identify a spelled word which he only partially recognized. While a score obtained by multiple choice has some uncertainty, the examiner may judge the range of uncertainty. One point is allowed for each correct recognition for a maximum score of eight points.

Word-picture Matching

This is the first subtest in which comprehension of the meaning of written words is involved. The ten words selected (on Card 5) correspond to objects, actions, colors, numbers and geometric forms appearing on Cards 2 and 3. These are the same words which were used earlier in the testing of auditory word discrimination, naming and oral word-reading. This task may be performed well by patients whose poor auditory comprehension has caused them to fail on the preceding pair of subtests. Understanding individual words is a prerequisite for comprehension of any written sentences. The highest intercorrelations of this subtest are within the cluster of reading tasks: .67 with Word Recognition, .66 with Sentences and Paragraphs and .63 with Symbol and Word Discrimination.

ADMINISTRATION AND SCORING. The test words are printed on Card 5, while the corresponding pictures to be identified are on Cards 2 and 3. Card 5 is slipped under the appropriate picture card in such a way that the edge of the picture-stimulus card acts as a line guide for each successive test word, and the subject is instructed to point to the picture (or number or color or form) corresponding to the word. Card 5 is slipped from Card 2 to Card 3 as called for by the location of the test picture. The score is based on one point per correct match for a maximum of ten.

Reading Sentences and Paragraphs

Some patients show an abrupt failure at the simplest levels of sentence comprehension, although they read well at the one-word level. As in the case of oral sentence-reading, we are dealing here with a complex task which is most difficult to predict from performances in other more elementary tasks. Hence, this subtest primarily serves the purpose of describing the level of functioning in an important linguistic skill, rather than pointing to an elementary component of language which may help explain more complex functions. Four of the five highest correlations with other subtests, ranging from .53 to .66, are within the reading cluster. There is a correlation of .67 with Primer-level Dictation.

The technique of sentence completion with a four-way multiple choice is easy to convey to the patient and much less subject to guesswork than the true-false question. The choice of possible answers always includes several wrong responses which are associatively related to words in the stimulus material. Thus, it is not possible to pass these questions merely by noting a salient word and selecting an associate to it. The range is from first-grade to high-school level difficulty in a ten-item scale.

ADMINISTRATION AND SCORING. Use Cards 12 through 16. Two buffer items are provided and the examiner may read one or both of these aloud, as he considers necessary, pointing to each of the choices in turn, for the patient to indicate his selection. Examiner underlines patient's choice in the test booklet. The first regular item is then administered without any help in the form of oral reading, although the examiner may, for impaired patients, point to the words in the test sentence and to the sequence of choices. One point is allowed for each correct answer for a maximum of ten points.

WRITING

The examination of writing is analogous to that of speech, in that we examine the mechanics of writing movements, the recall of written symbols for execution through various modes of stimulation and the formulation of connected material in free narrative and from dictation. These correspond to the levels of articulation, word-finding and formulation of connected discourse in speech.

Mechanics of Writing

The score for mechanics is in the form of a four-step rating scale, based on the writing (either to command, by transcription or by direct copy) of the patient's name and address and the "quick-brown-fox" sentence. While this aspect of writing is a prerequisite for the simplest propositional writing, no element of encoding ideas or even phonetic transcription is involved here; consequently, correlations with other parts of the battery are not high. The closest association is with Primer-level Dictation (correlation .55) and the next closest is with Word-picture Matching (.51), Spelling to Dictation (.48) and Written Confrontation Naming (.48).

ADMINISTRATION AND SCORING. The patient is instructed to write his name and address using his more able hand. If he fails, they are block printed by the examiner and patient is instructed to transcribe them into his own handwriting or, failing that, to copy them. The patient is then required to copy the printed sentence in the test booklet into his own handwriting or, if that is not possible, to copy in the same form. Performance is scored only with respect to the recall of the movements of letter formation, according to the following standards:

(3) Normal (making allowance for non-preferred hand)
(2) Partly illegible, but can form all letters in longhand by transcription or on command
(1) Fails some letters in transcription but can copy block-printing
(0) Few recognizable letters

Recall of Written Symbols

This subtest is divided into two separately scored sections: (1) *Serial Writing*—alphabet and numbers to 21 and (2) *Primer-level Dictation*—writing individual numbers, letters and primer words to dictation. This represents the easiest level of written symbol recall—a level which does not yet involve any communication of meaning. The association of the written response to the dictated stimulus does not necessarily imply the intermediation of comprehension. The two sections have an intercorrelation of .58. This relatively low value probably reflects the lack of association between serial symbol writing and other parts of the test battery; it is the highest correlation between serial writing and any other subtest. Primer-level Dictation correlates best (.67) with Reading Sentences and Paragraphs, but its next three highest correlations are within the writing cluster.

ADMINISTRATION AND SCORING. In part one, Serial Writing, the patient is instructed to write the alphabet and then to write numbers up to twenty-one. If he does not understand, the first three numbers of each set may be written to start him off. The score is the total number of different, correct letters and numbers, combined for a maximum score of 47. In part two, *Primer-level Dictation*, the letters, numbers and primer words in the test booklet are dictated and the score is the combined total correct (up to fifteen) from these three sets.

Written Word-finding

This subtest taps the written vocabulary beyond the primer level, in the range of words of average difficulty. It, too, is subdivided into two subsections: (1) *Spelling to Dictation* and (2) *Written Confrontation Naming*.

SPELLING TO DICTATION. Performance requires writing, oral spelling and the use of cutout anagrams. Spelling from dictation is theoretically possible without the intervention of the comprehension of meaning. Some individuals show a strongly automatized phonetic association between auditory input and spelled output. The value of anagrams as an alternative way of demonstrating writing ability is that it circumvents difficulties in the mechanics of writing, but not in letter

choice or ordering. Oral spelling, however, is partly autonomous from the written performance. Many individuals have the knack of rattling off oral spelling quite rapidly without much success in using this to guide their written spelling. Oral spelling calls on auditory-verbal imagery and purely temporal sequencing, aided by highly overlearned sequential probabilities among the letters of English words. This contrasts with the requirement of spatial sequencing in writing, and with the fact that the slowness of writing greatly reduces the benefits of overlearned temporal sequences in the motor-kinesthetic sphere.

The correlation of spelling with other subtests is highest within the writing cluster, .77 with Written Confrontation Naming and .67 with Sentences to Dictation.

Administration and scoring. The words are presented orally, with clear enunciation, and the patient is required to write them on a clean sheet of paper. The test may be discontinued at the discretion of the examiner if the patient is clearly beyond his depth. If there are any words failed in writing, the patient should be asked to spell them aloud and assemble them with anagrams. Present the anagram letters required for the word in a jumbled array with two extraneous letters included. Score written spelling only. Note additional success in oral spelling and anagrams for qualitative interpretation.

WRITTEN CONFRONTATION NAMING. This is the first subtest in which the patient is asked to convey information in writing. The vocabulary used consists of some of the objects, colors, forms, actions and numbers previously used to test auditory comprehension, naming and reading. In spite of the logical parallel between this and oral confrontation naming, the correlation between the two subtests is only .48. This test has its strongest intercorrelations within the writing cluster and secondary correlations in the reading comprehension group, .56 with Word-picture Matching and .53 with Reading Sentences and Paragraphs.

Administration and scoring. The examiner, using Cards 2 and 3, points *silently* to the items in the order they appear in the test booklet. The patient is given paper and pencil and instructed orally or in pantomime to write the names. Score one for each correctly spelled response, for a maximum of ten.

Written Formulation

In this subtest, we assess the patient's level of function in the complex task of writing connected sentences, first in free narrative about the "cookie theft" scene, then in response to dictation.

NARRATIVE WRITING. This performance is the complex resultant of the ability to find the needed words, to formulate sentences and to spell. Many patients who can write individual words well are overwhelmed by the task of forming sentences and give up after a feeble effort. Occasionally, one obtains fluent but grossly irrelevant writing, usually from patients who also produce fluent, paraphasic speech. The interplay of several diverse factors in this task results in low intercorrelations with other subtests. The highest correlation (.58) is with Written Confrontation Naming and the next two with Spelling to Dictation (.54) and Sentences to Dictation (.49).

Administration and scoring. The patient is given a fresh sheet of paper, presented with the "cookie theft" picture (Card 1) and instructed to, "Write as much as you can about what you see going on in this picture." He is encouraged to continue writing for two minutes, but may be permitted to work longer if his writing is relevant, but exceptionally slow. Adequacy is scored on a five-point scale from zero to four where:

0 = No relevant writing
1 = Isolated words or very small groupings

2 = Incomplete but relevant sentences
3 = Unduly simplified but correct sentences
4 = Full description in grammatical sentences

If writing is copious but paraphasic, the scoring standards should be applied to relevant words, if any, which are included in the production. Thus, fluent paraphasic sentences in which an occasional relevant word or phrase can be identified would be scored one. Those in which relevant statements are embedded in nonsentence form would be scored two; those in which sentences are complete and relevant but contaminated by paraphasia would score three.

SENTENCES TO DICTATION. While the relatively unstructured writing task of free narrative is beyond the capacity of most aphasics, many of them reveal potential ability when offered preformulated sentences from dictation. The three sentences provided refer to the "cookie theft" picture and are graded in length and grammatical complexity. This subtest has its highest correlation (.67) with Spelling to Dictation, and three of the next four most closely correlated tests are in the writing cluster.

Administration and scoring. The three sentences given in the test booklet are dictated, with no time limit imposed on the patient's writing. Each of the three sentences is scored from zero to four points according to the scale in the test booklet, and the subtest score is the total of the three, for a maximum of twelve. Insertion or substitution of irrelevant words is called "paragraphia" and is scored on a three-point scale as (0) conspicuous, (1) minor and (2) absent. This rating is based on the subtests, *Narrative Writing* and *Sentences to Dictation.*

Chapter 5

SUPPLEMENTARY LANGUAGE TESTS

We present here a number of further procedures for the use of the examiner who is interested in a more complete understanding of the patient's language functioning because of its value in diagnosis, therapy or both. These procedures consist of tests with which there is experimental or clinical experience, but which have not been incorporated into the aphasia battery. They cover an exploration of psycholinguistic factors in auditory comprehension and in expression, exploration of disorders of repetition, study of the sparing of comprehension of whole body movement commands and screening for hemispheric disconnection symptoms.

PSYCHOLINGUISTIC EXPLORATION OF AUDITORY COMPREHENSION

Goodglass, Gleason and Hyde (1970) presented evidence that impaired auditory comprehension cannot be regarded as an undifferentiated disorder, and that the relative impairment of vocabulary comprehension, span and prepositional comprehension varies systematically in diagnostic subgroups of patients. Their results are in accord with Luria's report (1966) that constructions (usually hinging on prepositions) which signal logico-grammatical relationships are impaired in certain forms of aphasia. These, among others, are covered by the items suggested in this section.

Prepositions of Location

Invert a cup on the table and give patient a penny. Sit alongside the patient to elim-

inate ambiguity about "front" and "back" of the cup. Say, "Put the penny *under* the cup. Put the penny *behind* the cup. Put the penny *to the left of* the cup. Put the penny *in front of* the cup. Put the penny *on* the cup. Hold the penny *over* the cup. Put the penny *to the right of* the cup." Place penny a few inches in front of the cup and say, "Move the penny *away* from the cup. Move the penny *toward* the cup." If there is any hesitancy or error, repeat the commands in random order until you can tell which are consistently passed, which are "brittle areas" and which are pure guesswork.

"Before"-"After"

Ask for a "yes"-"no" response to the following:
> "Do you eat lunch *after* supper?"
> "Do you eat supper *after* lunch?"
> "Do you put on your shoes *after* your stockings?"
> "Do you put on your stockings *before* your shoes?"
> "Is noontime *before* evening?"
> "Is evening *before* noontime?"

"With-to" Pointing

In commands involving manipulation of one object to touch another, the patient may tend to pick up the first object named, regardless of the prepositions "with" and "to" which may tell him to do otherwise.

In the following series, we begin with a buffer item to create the proper performance set, and then use a number of elongated

41

objects (comb, pencil, scissors, knife, fork, cigarette) with commands.

Buffer: Place the comb and pencil (or any other pair) on the table and say, "Pick up the comb. Now touch the pencil with the comb." Remove the first two objects and put down any two others (e.g., spoon and scissors). Say, "Touch the scissors with the spoon." Then, "With the spoon, touch the scissors." Continue replacing the objects with a different pair after each item, being careful to randomize the left or right position of the object to be picked up so as to control for consistent lateral preferences. Give commands in the format:

"Touch the _____ with the _____."
"With the _____ touch the _____."

Passive Subject-Object Discrimination

The passive word order (e.g., "The lion was killed by the tiger") reverses the position of agent vs. victim, with respect to the word order expected in the more common active sentence construction. The listener must utilize the particles "was" and "by" to identify agent and victim. Our data indicate this to be a most difficult discrimination for aphasics, who often interpret the sentence on the basis of the active word order, namely that the agent precedes the verb and the victim follows. In order to examine the comprehension of the passive construction, we present the following:

"If I tell you, 'The lion was killed by the tiger,' which animal is dead?"

"If I tell you, 'The lion was killed by the tiger,' which animal killed the other one?"

"If I tell you, 'The boy was slapped by the girl,' which one slapped the other? Which one felt the slap?"

"If I tell you, 'The car was damaged by the motorcycle,' which vehicle needs repair?"

If the patient is unable to produce the necessary one-word answers, the administra-

tion may be adapted to "yes-no" form. Thus, in the first item the examiner may ask, "Does this mean the lion is dead?" or "Does this mean the lion did the killing?"

Comprehension of Possessive Relationship

One of the most difficult tasks for some patients is the comprehension of the relationship between two nouns which is symbolized by the possessive "s." This difficulty is highlighted when the semantic structure does not contribute to the interpretation. That is, "my sister's hat" is a semantically nonreversible relationship, which is understandable even without the "s." When both nouns are humans, however, as in "my sister's father," the weight of the discrimination falls entirely on the word order. Thus, in order to test this feature, we present the following task to the patient:

"Suppose I point to someone across the street (examiner points) and say 'That person is my wife's brother.' Am I looking at a man or a woman?" (Or, "Is that person a man? . . . Is it a woman?")

Repeat this procedure for "my sister's husband," "my uncle's daughter," "my son's wife."

PSYCHOLINGUISTIC EXPLORATION OF EXPRESSION

The breakdown of grammatical performance in aphasia is manifested chiefly by the unavailability of syntactic constructions, apart from the simplest and most stereotyped. At more severe levels, articles, auxiliary verbs, prepositions and inflectional endings are lost, especially those which occur as the first, unstressed word in a sentence. Attempts to elicit these difficulties by means of structured tasks sometimes lead to performances that are at odds with spontaneous production. That is, a patient whose spontaneous speech is agrammatic may repeat short sentences of all types well, while a grammatically fluent patient does poorly. Therefore, these formal tasks should be considered in their own right and compared with the impression gained by listening to free conversation.

Both repetition and sentence-manipulation tasks are used, since these structured test procedures permit exploring for competence with forms which may not have occurred in free conversation. Included in the sentence-repetition tasks are constructions with a preponderance of "small grammatical words," since these have proven empirically very difficult for patients with "conduction aphasia," a selective disorder of repetition.

Repetition Tasks

CONTRAST BETWEEN INDICATIVE AND INTERROGATIVE.
1. The man works here.
2. Does the man work here?
3. He can swim a mile.
4. Can he swim a mile?
5. He is very rich.
6. Is he very rich?
7. He sells cars.
8. Does he sell cars?
9. She ought to go.
10. Ought she to go?

CONDITIONAL CONSTRUCTION.
1. If she cries, feed her.
2. If he moves, shoot.
3. If it rains, stay home.
4. Feed her if she cries.
5. Shoot if he moves.
6. Stay home if it rains.

Manipulation of Verb Tense

The agrammatic patient works with a reduced repertory of verbal endings, often having only the verb stem and the "-ing" form at his disposal. Free conversation sometimes fails to give a complete sampling of his abilities with tenses, as there may be little or no reference to past or future events. Consequently, sentence-completion tests along the lines of the following are useful to find out if the patient can adjust the verb tense to past and future, following the semantic demands of the sentence.

"The baby cries every night. She did the same last night.
Last night, the baby (what?)."

"John swims every Sunday. Next Sunday, he will do the same.
Next Sunday, he (what?)."

"I work every evening and tomorrow I will do the same.
Tomorrow night, I (what?)."

Asking Questions

"YES"-"NO" QUESTIONS. These questions begin with an initial unstressed auxiliary verb, either a form of "do" or a modal ("can," "may") followed by the subject and principal verb. This task is extremely difficult for the Broca's aphasic but is usually performed easily by Wernicke's aphasics.

"How would you ask me if it's raining?"
"How would you ask me if I have the time?"
"How would you ask a jeweler if he fixes clocks?"
"How would you ask a stranger if he speaks English?"
"How would you ask a little boy if he can write his name?"

"WH"-QUESTIONS. These are questions opening with interrogative pronouns or adverbs, such as, "who," "where," "how," "what" and "why." While the initial word is always followed by an inversion of the subject-verb sequence, this form of question is easier than the "yes"-"no" form, perhaps because it begins with a stressed word. To elicit questions in this form, the following stimuli may be used:

"How would you ask me what the weather is like outside?"
"How would you ask me the time?"
"How would you ask a salesman the price of a certain hat?"
"How would you ask where the bus stops?'
"How would you ask to find out the owner of a certain car?"

Repetition Tasks for Conduction Aphasia

The characteristic features of this disorder, aside from difficulty with the repetition of small grammatical words, is the predominance of literal paraphasia (transposition and substitution of phonemes) in all but number words. In the case of numbers, the errors take the form of verbal paraphasia (substitution of other numbers).

REPETITION OF DIFFICULT WORDS.
   Baseball player
   Peanut butter
   Pussy willow
   Methodist Episcopal
REPETITION WITH GRAMMATICAL WORDS.
   One would have been enough.
   He asked where he was when we were
      there.
   No ifs, ands, or buts.*
REPETITION OF NUMBERS AND NUMBER-WORD COMBINATIONS. (Note contrast between verbal paraphasia on numbers and literal paraphasia on nonnumber words.)
   Fifty-seven
   Eight forty-six
   Forty-eight divided by sixteen
   Three-quarters equal seventy-five percent

TESTS FOR
DISCONNECTION SYNDROMES

Dissociation of Modalities in Naming

Confrontation naming is almost always at the same level of adequacy, regardless of whether the object is presented visually, by touch or by producing its characteristic sound. Rare exceptions to this rule are found, and these exceptions are likely to involve the interruption of fibers bringing sensory information from the right cerebral hemisphere to the left, where they must be received in order to activate a verbal response.

* This item, introduced by Dr. Norman Geschwind, has almost invariably baffled conduction aphasics.

Naming by Touch in Either Hand

Use a collection of small objects (coin, pencil, key, eyeglasses, comb, paper clip, ring). Subject is required to keep his eyes shut, while each object is presented to the left hand to be palpated and named. In a different sequence, they are presented to the right hand for naming. If there is variability of success, repeat the series in random order of presentation until it is clear whether one hand is superior to the other. Clear inferiority of the left hand raises the presumption that there is an interruption of the sensory information from the right hemisphere on its way to the left, where it must be received in order to activate a verbal response. Such an interruption involves fibers in, or going through, the corpus callosum. Tactile naming may be affected by loss of touch and position sense, i.e., a primary sensory defect. Such a primary sensory defect is established if the patient fails to match objects tactually with his left hand (using multiple-choice presentation).

Minor Hand Agraphia

Just as incoming sensory information from the minor hemisphere may be disconnected from the language system, a similar disconnection may prevent the outflow of language-related motor instructions necessary for writing with the nonpreferred hand. A disorder of this nature can be inferred only if writing is retained to at least a moderate degree in the preferred hand. If the right hand is paralyzed, reading and oral spelling may be used as a test of the functioning of the written language system. If these functions are intact, then agraphia of the minor hand would again signify failure of transmission of linguistically organized motor instructions across the corpus callosum.

Chapter 6

SUPPLEMENTARY NONLANGUAGE TESTS

The study of defects associated with aphasia has identified a number of higher perceptual-motor performances which are not strictly within the sphere of language, but which, like language, are vulnerable to injuries lateralized on one side or the other and, in some cases, highly localizable within a hemisphere. This section presents an examination procedure for the major parietal lobe cluster, consisting of tests for constructional apraxia, finger agnosia, acalculia and right-left confusion. Normative data for aphasic patients are presented in Table 5. In addition, we present an apraxia examination covering buccofacial praxis, limb praxis, whole body movements and serial actions with objects. The latter examination is evaluated clinically by the examiner, rather than with reference to statistical norms, which are lacking.

There are other localizing specific deficits, not covered by these test procedures. A partial list would include visual agnosia, auditory agnosia, agnosia for faces (prosopagnosia) and the minor hemisphere symptoms of left-sided neglect of personal and extrapersonal space and dressing apraxia. For discussion of these disorders, the reader is referred to Critchley (1966).

THE PARIETAL LOBE BATTERY

Constructional Apraxia

This refers to a deficit in the execution of visuo-spatial tasks, as in drawing, assembling stick designs and constructing three-dimen-sional block arrangements. Constructional abilities are somewhat vulnerable to injuries in any part of the cortex, but the most severe disorganization of these efforts is associated with parietal lobe injury. While either left or right parietal damage may produce severe deficits in construction, there are more dramatic failures with right-sided damage and total failure with bilateral parietal lobe damage.

Table 5. Range, Mean and Standard Deviation of Aphasics on Each Subtest

	N	Range	M	SD
Draw (Command)	139	0–13	7.4	3.7
Draw (Copy)	144	0–13	9.6	3.2
Stick Memory	137	0–14	7.4	3.8
Finger Comprehension	133	3–48	37.2	13.0
Finger-naming	118	0–32	16.8	12.8
Visual Finger-matching	108	3–40	33.9	8.9
Tactile Fingers	133	0–32	24.7	7.8
Total Fingers	107	0–152	113.8	34.4
Right-left	135	0–16	11.0	4.6
Arithmetic	146	0–31	15.2	9.5
Clock-setting	146	0–12	9.0	3.1
Blocks (3-D)	133	0–10	6.1	3.3

Constructional difficulties in this battery are sampled by three subtests.

    Drawing to command
    Stick construction (memory)
    Three-dimensional blocks

DRAWING TO COMMAND. The patient is required to draw each of the following to command on a blank sheet of paper, receiving up to three points credit on the first item and up to two points on the remaining five, for a total possible score of thirteen.

This subtest correlates best with 3-D Block Construction (.58) and next best with Stick Construction Memory (.48).

Clock

Instruction: "Draw the *face of a clock* showing the numbers and the two hands."
Score: 0 to 3. One point each for:
Approximately circular face
Symmetry of number placement
Correctness of numbers

Daisy

Instruction: "Draw a *daisy*."
Score: 0 to 2. One point each for:
General shape—center with petals around
    it
Symmetry of petal arrangement

Elephant

Instruction: "Draw an *elephant*."
Score: 0 to 2. One point each for:
General shape (legs, trunk, head, body)
Relative proportions correct

Cross

Instruction: "You know what the *Red Cross* looks like? Draw an outline of it without taking your pencil off the paper."
Score: 0 to 2. One point each for:
Basic configuration
Ability to form all corners adequately
    with a continuous line

Cube

Instruction: "Draw a *cube-shaped block* in perspective, as it would look if you could see the top and two sides."
Score: 0 to 2. One point each for:
Grossly correct attempt
Correctness of perspective

House

Instruction: "Draw a *house* in perspective, so you can see the roof and two sides."
Score: 0 to 2. One point each for:

Grossly correct features of house
Accuracy of perspective

Models for copying each of the above should be provided by the examiner. It is of interest to see if copying is much better than drawing to command without a model. Drawing to command and from a model were

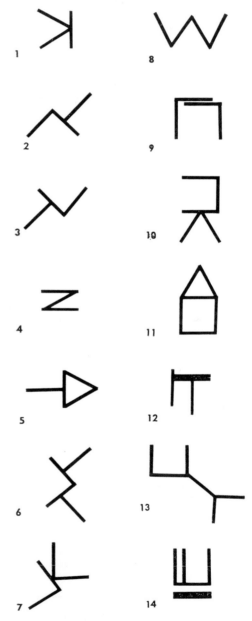

FIGURE 3. Stick test figures.

strongly correlated (.78) with both loaded about equally on the Parietal Lobe Factor (II).   Score only Drawing to Command.

This subtest correlates best with 3-D Block Construction (.58) and next best with Stick Construction Memory (.48).

STICK CONSTRUCTION MEMORY.   Matchstick geometric figures have long been used in informal clinical tests of constructional ability.   They are discussed by Goldstein and Scheerer (1941) who also published a test using plastic sticks.   The present version differs in two ways from the Goldstein-Scheerer test.   First, it is shorter and graduated more steeply in difficulty, to tap the normal range of ability.   Secondly, while three items (W and Z-shaped figures, and a house-shaped figure) may be encoded in memory as a familiar unit (=Goldstein's "concrete"), our interest was not in contrasting codable vs. noncodable, but in scaling constructional ability.

The materials consist of twelve wooden sticks one-quarter-inch square by three

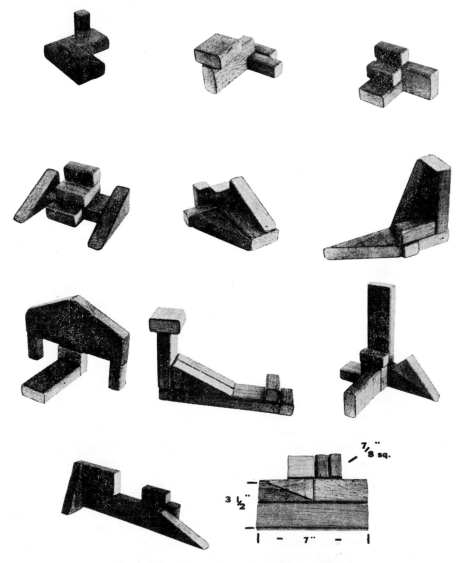

FIGURE 4.   Three-dimensional block designs.

inches long, six for the examiner's demonstrations and six for the patient.

Each of the fourteen designs in Figure 3 is first assembled before the patient by the examiner, who instructs the patient to watch closely since he will be expected to make the same designs. After the design has been exposed for ten seconds, it is swept up and the patient is given the signal to reproduce it.

Score is based on one point per correct item. Every stick must be in its position for credit to be allowed, although minor inaccuracies in the size of angles need not be penalized.

THREE-DIMENSIONAL BLOCKS. Three-dimensional block construction has the highest intercorrelations of any of the subtests within the parietal lobe test cluster. The five highest are with Right-left Discrimination (.66), Clock-setting (.65), Sticks (.60), Arithmetic (.59) and Drawing to Command (.58). There are no correlations over .50 with language subtests.

The materials consist of miniature kindergarten blocks. The dimensions of the blocks and the photographs of the ten three-dimensional constructions presented for the patient to reproduce, appear in Figure 4. Up to one minute is allowed for each construction and complete accuracy of placement is required for credit—one point per item.

Finger Agnosia

Finger recognition is normally performed with few or no errors except by patients with lesions of the major parietal lobe. This test is considerably more selective, in this respect, than the constructional tests. Defects may appear in naming or in finger-name comprehension, in visual-visual or visual-tactile matching. The present subtest samples all modalities with an extensive (152 point) survey. However, this is so arranged that credit is allowed for easy items if more difficult ones are passed, greatly economizing the time required for the test. This subtest correlates best with Arithmetic (.58), 3-D Blocks (.57) and Stick Construc-

tion (.52) and has a loading of .74 on the Parietal Lobe Factor (II).

Materials consist of drawings of a left and a right hand, palm down, and a hand-shielding box (Figure 5) which are used for the visual-tactile matching subset.

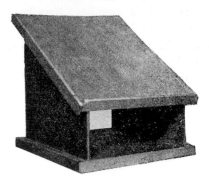

FIGURE 5.   Box-shield used for tactile-visual finger-matching.

Prior to testing, rings are removed from patient's fingers, in order to eliminate cues as to the "ring finger," and the examiner reviews the standard names: "thumb," "index," "middle," "ring" and "little" finger. Because of the greater sensitivity to confusion found among the middle three fingers, the following weighting of scores is applied in all subsections of the test: three middle fingers—two points each; thumb and little finger—one point each.

VERBAL.

1. *Comprehension.*

a. *Picture hand.*

TRIAL A. Place drawing with fingers oriented to patient. Instruct patient to indicate which finger you name. If no errors are made, allow full credit on Trial B and on Part b—own hand. Each finger is sampled twice, randomizing order of presentation.

TRIAL B. (Omit with credit if Trial A is perfect.) Place drawing with fingers oriented away from patient and proceed as in Trial A. Score for each trial, zero to sixteen.

b. *Own hand.* (Omit and credit if either Trial A or Trial B is perfectly performed.) Examiner names and patient indicates corresponding finger of either hand. Same sequence and scoring as in preceding tests.

2. *Finger-naming* (using picture).

TRIAL A. Picture oriented with fingers toward patient. Each finger is pointed to twice in random order for patient to name, with a total possible score of sixteen. Omit Trial B with full credit if no errors are made on Trial A.

TRIAL B. Same as Trial A, with fingers oriented away from patient.

VISUAL-VISUAL.

1. *Paired-finger identification.* Patient's left (or nonhemiplegic) hand is placed on table and drawing of picture hand is oriented at right angles to it. Patient is instructed to move or point to the two fingers of his hand corresponding to those which examiner touches simultaneously on the drawing.

Score: Allow two points per item; no partial credit.

Sequence for paired-finger identification:

thumb-little_____   thumb-index _____
middle-ring _____   ring-little_____
index-little _____   index-middle_____
thumb-middle_____   thumb-ring _____
index-ring _____   middle-little _____
                      Subscore (0–20) ___

2. *Matching two-finger positions.* Examiner holds up pairs of fingers, dorsal side to patient, asking patient to copy the gesture with the same fingers. Follow the same sequence as in paired-finger identification.

TACTILE-VISUAL. Patient inserts hand into box-shield, on upper surface of which is placed the picture of the hand corresponding to the hand being tested. Examiner touches each finger twice in random order and patient points it out on the picture. Each hand should be tested unless there is no tactile sensation in one hand. Using a scoring system of two points for the three middle fingers and one point for the thumb and little fingers, the maximum score for both hands is thirty-two. (Box-shield is illustrated in Figure 5.)

SUMMARY OF POSSIBLE SCORES.

Verbal

1. Comprehension
    a. Picture hand   0–32
    b. Own hand   0–16
2. Finger-naming   0–32
                                    Subtotal   80

Visual-visual

1. Paired-finger identification   0–20
2. Matching two-finger positions   0–20
                                    Subtotal   40

Tactile-visual   0–32
                                    Subtotal   32
                                    Total possible 152

Acalculia

Disturbances of calculation are not exclusive to parietal lobe injury. The memory and mental manipulations that are required suffer from brain damage of many types. However, very severe loss of number sense and of the principles of arithmetic operations (especially when reinforced by deficits in finger recognition and right-left orientation) are more indicative of selective parietal lesions than is a general lowering of scores.

When the patient confuses the columns in addition or subtraction, but preserves the individual numerical operations, one may suspect the spatial confusion associated with right parietal damage. Aphasic patients may misname numbers as they write them. In some cases, they go on to a correct written solution in spite of their paraphasic sidetalk but, in some cases, they are diverted by their misnaming and carry out operations on the erroneously spoken numbers.

ARITHMETIC. The arithmetic subtest correlates best with 3-D Blocks (.59), Finger Recognition (.58) and Right-left Discrimination (.53). A correlation of .53 was also obtained with Phonetic Word-matching—the only correlation of over .50 outside of the parietal lobe test cluster. Its loading on Factor II is .60.

The following items of progressive complexity are given for solution with paper and pencil.

Addition

3	11	14	16	12	96	589	273
+5	+8	+13	+27	45	53	234	491
				+32	28	+163	587
					+17		+169

Subtraction

8	17	16	29	52	549	352	500
−5	−4	−8	−16	−25	−138	−269	−349

Multiplication

$2 \times 3 =$	$3 \times 6 =$	$8 \times 7 =$	12	23	214	358
			×3	×12	×35	×679

Division

$$2\sqrt{6} \qquad 4\sqrt{16} \qquad 8\sqrt{168} \qquad 7\sqrt{434} \qquad 9\sqrt{621} \qquad 25\sqrt{150}$$

$$14\sqrt{161} \qquad\qquad 68\sqrt{22100} \qquad\qquad 489\sqrt{27384}$$

Answers

Addition	Subtraction	Multiplication	Division
8	3	6	3
19	13	18	4
27	8	56	21
43	13	36	62
89	27	276	69
194	411	7,490	6
986	83	243,082	$11\frac{1}{2}$
1,520	151		325
			56

One point each, score: 0–32

CLOCK-SETTING. While clock-setting logically entails a sense of number relations, it also brings into play geometric representation. On both counts, it is sensitive to parietal lobe damage. In our sample, Clock-setting correlated as highly with two auditory comprehension subtests (.55 with Word Discrimination, .60 with Commands) as with subtests of the parietal lobe cluster. Within the latter group, it is correlated with 3-D Blocks (.59), Stick Construction (.58), Right-left Discrimination (.57) and Arithmetic (.52).

Clock-setting is administered by showing the patient a sheet on which four blank clock faces are drawn, with only short lines marking the positions of the twelve numbers. The patient is asked to draw in the two hands of the clock to make the faces read 1:00, 3:00, 9:15 and 7:30. Scoring is based on one point for the correct placement of each hand plus one point for indicating correctly the relative lengths of the hour and minute hands, allowing three points per item and a zero-to-twelve point range for this subtest.

Right-left Orientation

Right-left discrimination is one of the four components of Gerstmann's syndrome, along with finger agnosia, calculation disorder and agraphia—the constellation being a strong indicator of a lesion of the left angular gyrus at the posterior temporo-parietal junction. In the present battery, Right-left orientation correlates best with 3-D Blocks (.66), Clock-setting (.57), Arithmetic (.56) and Finger Recognition (.47). It has no correlations of over .50 in the aphasia test proper. It is not one of the subtests most strongly loaded on the Parietal Lobe Factor (II), having a loading of only .47.

The following commands are presented, with the most difficult given first and, if passed, credit allowed for all remaining items. If the first two items of any group are failed, skip to the next easier level. Score one point for a correct response, half credit

if correct but preceded by hesitation (maximum score is sixteen).

Double-other person.
(Crossed)* Point with your right hand to my right shoulder.
(Uncrossed) Point with your left hand to my right eye.
(Crossed) Point with your left hand to my left hand.
(Uncrossed) Point with your right hand to my left ear.
Double-own body. (Eyes shut—full credit; eyes open—half credit.)
(Crossed) Put your left hand on your right ear.
(Uncrossed) Put your right hand on your right eye.
(Crossed) Put your right hand on your left shoulder.
(Uncrossed) Put your left hand on your left ear.
Single-other person.
Show me my right hand.
Show me my left shoulder.
Show me my left ear.
Show me my right eye.
Single-self. (Eyes shut—full credit; eyes open—half credit.)
Show me your right hand.
Show me your left eye.
Show me your left shoulder.
Show me your right ear.

Since the test is given orally, allowance must be made for auditory comprehension difficulty of aphasic patients. In order to be considered significantly depressed, the z-score value for right-left discrimination should be lower than that for the Body-part Identification subtest.

APRAXIA

Apraxia refers to the loss of capacity to carry out purposeful movements, when

* Requires patient to cross the midline of his body.

motor strength and coordination are adequate. When apraxia is severe, it takes the form of ineptness in manipulating everyday objects. More often, it is milder, and is expressed in the inability to carry out pretended movements on request, while having an actual object at hand is a cue for normal motor behavior in using it.

The hierarchical relationship between pretended actions to command and those determined by concrete contextual cues is observed in most cases, with performance to imitation lying between them in difficulty. However, it is not clear whether this sequence of difficulty is universal.

Apraxia may affect movements of the face and bucco-respiratory apparatus, autonomously from limb movements. Limb apraxia is commonly bilateral although paralysis of one side may obscure it. Except for "dressing apraxia," these movement disorders are overwhelmingly associated with lesions of the left hemisphere and are, therefore, commonly associated with aphasia. However, there does not appear to be a psychological causal relationship between apraxia and aphasia, since they vary independently as to presence and severity. The lesions of apraxia generally lie within the same gross brain areas as those causing aphasia. The precise relation between apractic symptom and lesion localization has not been as well established as the corresponding relationships for language disturbance. For a proposed theory of localization, the reader is referred to Geschwind (1965).

For the examination outlined below, there are as yet no norms. Previous experience (Goodglass and Kaplan, 1963) shows that raters agree very well on judgments of "normal," "partially adequate" and "failed."

Particular features of interest are the following:

Body-part As Object (BPO)

Apraxic patients have a strong tendency to represent the use of an implement by making the hand or finger take the role of the implement and come into contact with the object of the action. Thus, the index finger rubbed against the teeth becomes the toothbrush in response to, "Show me how you would pretend to brush your teeth with a toothbrush." The fist pounded on a surface becomes the hammer in response to, "Show me how you would pretend to hammer a nail."

This behavior is the rule up to age eight (Kaplan, 1968), but is quite rare in normal adults. When a patient performs in this way, he should be instructed to try again as though he were really holding the implement in his hand. If this does not modify the performance, the examiner demonstrates and invites the patient to imitate. The ability to correct performance on verbal instructions is counterindicative of apraxia, while the inability to change even after demonstration is typical of the apraxic patient.

Verbalizing Instead of Performing Buccal Commands

Patients with bucco-facial apraxia, in response to instructions to "cough" or "blow," sometimes explosively utter the name of the action in their effort to carry it out, even repeating this performance after demonstration by the examiner. This occurs only with performances that require the activation of the oral-respiratory apparatus.

Apraxia Test

Movements to Oral Command	Movements to Imitation	Movements with Real Object
Bucco-facial		
1. Cough	If failed to command	Does not apply
2. Sniff	If failed to command	If failed to command
3. Blow out a match	If failed to command	If failed to command
4. Suck through a straw	If failed to command	If failed to command
5. Puff out cheeks	If failed to command	Does not apply
Intransitive Limb		
1. Wave good-bye	If failed to command	Does not apply
2. Beckon "come here"	If failed to command	Does not apply
3. Finger on lip for "shsh"	If failed to command	Does not apply
4. Salute	If failed to command	Does not apply
5. Signal "stop"	If failed to command	Does not apply
*Transitive Limb**		
1. Brush teeth	If failed to command	If failed to command
2. Shave	If failed to command	If failed to command
3. Hammer	If failed to command	If failed to command
4. Saw board	If failed to command	If failed to command
5. Use screwdriver	If failed to command	If failed to command
Whole Body		
1. How does a boxer stand?	If failed to command	Does not apply
2. How does a golfer stand?	If failed to command	Does not apply
3. How does a soldier march in place?	If failed to command	Does not apply
4. How do you shovel snow?	If failed to command	Does not apply
5. Stand up, turn around twice and sit down.	If failed to command	Does not apply

Serial Actions (with real objects only)

1. Provide box of matches and pack of cigarettes.
   "Take a cigarette and light up."
2. Provide paper, envelope and penny stamp.
   "Put the paper in the envelope, seal it and stamp it."
3. Provide candle, candlestick, box of matches.
   "Put the candle in the holder, light it and blow it out."

* In items 2–5, for female subjects, say, "How would a man..."

Chapter 7

MAJOR APHASIC SYNDROMES AND ILLUSTRATIONS OF TEST PATTERNS

The various component elements in language disturbance, described in detail in Chapter 2, are not all free to appear in any combination or in isolation from each other. The clustering of these symptoms is, in part, a function of the anatomical organization of the language substrate in the brain. Equally important in determining the makeup of the syndromes is the fact that the locations of natural lesions—particularly cerebrovascular ones—tend to congregate in certain vulnerable areas of the brain.

The typology presented here is that which has had the widest currency in the world literature on aphasia since the end of the nineteenth century. The anatomical rationale for this typology dates back to Lichtheim's scheme which has been described in detail by Freud (1953). In spite of many innovations in nomenclature (Head, Luria, Wepman), the principal features of the various syndromes are described by each writer. The following presentation includes the alternative terms which have been applied.

FLUENCY VS. NONFLUENCY

The major subdivision among the aphasic syndromes is based on the character of the speech output. When the prerolandic (anterior) portion of the anatomic speech area (Broca's area) is involved, the flow of speech is more or less impaired at the levels of speech initiation, finding and sequencing of articulatory movements and production of grammatical sequences. The resulting speech —interrupted, awkwardly articulated with great effort—is referred to as "nonfluent." The contrasting or "fluent" forms of aphasia are marked by facility in articulation and many long runs of words in a variety of grammatical constructions, in conjunction with word-finding difficulty for substantives and picturable action words. The criteria for distinguishing between fluent and nonfluent aphasias are essentially those dealt with in the rating scale of speech characteristics (Chapter 4). The fluent aphasias are usually due to lesions posterior to the rolandic fissure, sparing Broca's area. Within this region, there is considerable variation in the detailed symptomatology of fluent aphasia. This variation is at least partly understandable in terms of the site of the injury. The significant variable components are the amount and type of paraphasia, auditory receptive loss, word-finding difficulty and impaired repetition.

Broca's Aphasia

(Head—"Verbal Aphasia"; Goldstein—"Motor Aphasia"; Luria—"Efferent Motor Aphasia"; Weisenburg and McBride—"Expressive Aphasia.")

We revert to the classical eponym rather than using the term "motor" aphasia or "expressive" aphasia, in order to avoid suggesting that speech output is normal in other forms of aphasia. Broca's aphasia is the common "anterior," or "nonfluent," aphasia depending on a lesion involving the third frontal convolution of the left hemisphere. Its essential characteristics are awkward articulation, restricted vocabulary, restriction of grammar to the simplest, most overlearned forms, and relative preservation of auditory comprehension. Written language follows the pattern of speech in that writing is usually at least as severely impaired as speech, while reading is only mildly affected.

At the early, severe levels, the patient may have lost even "yes" and "no" and be unable to initiate articulatory movements or to repeat any word. Nonspeech oral movements are often, *but not always,* affected. The variability of this association indicates that the articulatory failure is not caused by difficulty with oral movements per se. Comprehension of single words is prompt, but the patient may be confused by more complex spoken messages. As he begins to recover, the effortful, short-phrased quality of his speech is prominent. While a few difficult sounds may be simplified (e.g., "ts" for "ch"; "p" for "pl"), the articulatory difficulty is much reduced in imitation and may disappear in the recitation of memorized series. Thus, articulation is best judged during free conversation. Here, in addition to awkwardness and distortion of phonemes, we often hear some transpositions of phonemes as in "pelsil" for "pencil."

At the beginning of the recovery stage, too, object-naming often returns to functional levels, while syntax remains primitive. The patient may have only one- or two-word sentences and show his maximum difficulty in combining subject and verb, so that subject-noun phrase and verb phrase are produced as separate utterances. While he may try to form complete sentences, he has usually lost the ability to evoke syntactic patterns, and even a sentence repetition task may prove impossible from the grammatical point of view.

CONFIGURATION OF TEST SCORES. The Broca's aphasic, because of the sparsity and effort of his speech, is usually rated as "severe," i.e., level 1 or 2 on the severity

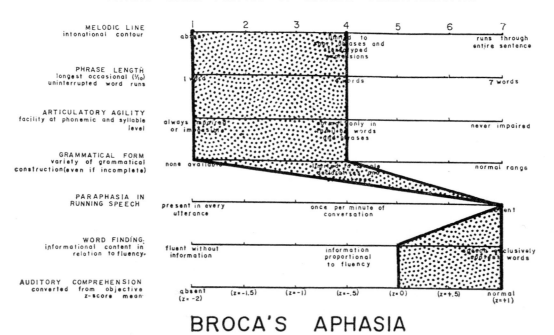

FIGURE 6.   Range of speech profile ratings characteristic of Broca's aphasia.

rating scale. Level 3, however, is not uncommon as the patient continues to recover. Those Broca's aphasic patients who go on to become only mild or residual aphasics (levels 4 and 5) lose the distinctive characteristics of Broca's aphasia. Their articulation and fluency approach normal levels and they show only some word-finding difficulty, making them barely distinguishable from mild anomic aphasics. However they never show the pressure of rapid speech or the blatant circumlocution and emptiness of substantive content which marks the *typical* anomic aphasic.

Figure 6 shows the range of ratings on the Profile of Speech Characteristics, consistent with Broca's aphasia.

The Aphasia Test z-score profile would show the fluency and severity scores lower than the auditory comprehension and naming

moderately depressed but quite cooperative. During his stay in the aphasia unit, he displayed considerable artistic talent but his poor morale prevented his following through with plans for formal art training. On a follow-up visit after six months at home, his speech showed essentially the same pattern described here, but with easier access to vocabulary. His spirits were greatly improved; he had become engaged to a hometown girl and made plans to enter art school.

During the initial interview his speech was limited to one-word answers, almost all nouns. The one verb used during the "cookie theft" picture narrative is uninflected, although it refers to a present progressive action. The interview required much questioning and guessing by the examiner. A sample of his production follows:

Interviewer	*Patient*
What did you do before you went to Vietnam?	Forces.
You were in the army?	Special forces. (poor articulation)
What did you do?	Boom!
I don't understand.	'Splosions.
(Further questioning by examiner)	Me...one guy.
Were you alone when you were injured?	Recon...scout.
What happened; why are you here?	Speech.
What happened?	Mortar.
(On presentation of "cookie theft" picture for description)	"Cookie jar...fall over...chair...water...empty...ov...ov...(examiner: "overflow?")
	Yeah.

scores. Oral reading and repetition would both be on a par with severity. The paraphasia pattern might show some literal paraphasia, but little of the other varieties. Reading comprehension is typically among the highest of the score clusters, writing among the lowest.

A CASE OF BROCA'S APHASIA. J.M. was a twenty-one-year-old, right-handed male with a tenth-grade education, wounded, nine months prior to his examination, by a mortar shell fragment which penetrated the frontoparietal region and left him with a severe right hemiplegia and a severe Broca's aphasia. At the time of examination, he was

The patient was rated at severity level "1," indicating that much questioning and inference were needed, with the interviewer carrying the burden of conversation.

Examination of the z-score profile (Figure 7) shows the typical pattern for Broca's aphasics. Fluency, including articulation is low, the severity rating is at "1," but auditory comprehension is little impaired. The naming cluster is decidedly superior to the fluency level. Paraphasia is virtually absent. Reading shows only mild impairment, except for the comprehension of oral spelling. While the recall of writing movements is good, the rest of writing performance is

Z-SCORE PROFILE OF APHASIA SUBSCORES

NAME: J.M.   DATE OF EXAM: 12-9-68

	-2.5	-2	-1	0	+1	+2	+2.5

SEVERITY RATING 0 1 2 3 4 5

FLUENCY
Artic. Rating — 1 2 3 4 5 6 7
Phrase Length — 1 2 3 4 5 6 7
Verbal Agility — 0 2 4 6 8 10 12 14

AUDITORY COMPREH.
Word Discrimin. — 15 20 25 30 35 40 45 50 55 60 65 70 72
Body Part Ident. — 5 10 15 20
Commands — 0 5 10
Complex Material — 0 2 4 6 8 10 12

NAMING
Responsive Naming — 0 5 10 15 20 25 30
Confront. Naming — 5 15 25 35 45 55 65 75 85 95 105
Animal Naming — 0 2 4 6 8 10 12 14 16 18 20 23
Body Part Naming — 0 5 10 15 20 25 30

ORAL READING
Word Reading — 0 5 10 15 20 25 30
Oral Sentence — 0 2 4 6 8 10

REPETITION
Repetition (wds.) — 0 2 4 6 8 10
Hi Prob. — 0 2 4 6 8
Lo Prob. — 0 2 4 6 8

PARAPHASIA
Neolog. — 2 4 6 8 10 12
Literal — 2 4 6 8 10 12 14 16
Verbal — 0 2 4 6 8 10 12 14 16 18 20 22 24
Extended — 2 4 6 8 10 12 14 16

AUTOM. SPEECH
Autom. Sequences — 0 2 4 6 8
Reciting — 0 2

READING COMPREH.
Symbol Discrim. — 4 6 8
Word Recog. — 2 4 6 8
Compr. Oral Spell. — 0 4 6 8
Wd. Picture Match — 0 2 4 6 8
Read. Sent. Parag. — 0 2 4 6 8 10

WRITING
Mechanics — 0 1 2
Serial Writing — 0 5 10 15 20 25 30 35 40 45 47
Primer. Dict. — 0 2 4 6 8 10 12 14 15
Writ. Confront. Naming — 0 2 4 6 8 10
Spelling To Dict. — 3 5 7 9 10
Sentences To Dict. — 2 4 6 8 10 12
Narrative Writ. — 1 2 3 4

MUSIC
Singing — 0 1 2
Rhythm — 0 1 2

PARIETAL
Drawing to Command — 1 3 5 7 9 11
Stick Memory — 1 3 5 7 9 11 14
Total Fingers — 40 60 80 100 120 140
Right-Left — 0 2 4 6 8 10 12 16
Arithmetic — 0 4 8 12 16 20 24 28 32
Clock Setting — 1 2 3 4 5 6 7 8 9 10 11 12
3 Dim. Blocks — 0 1 2 3 4 5 6 7 8 10

	-2.5	-2	-1	0	+1	+2	+2.5

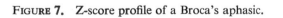

FIGURE 7. Z-score profile of a Broca's aphasic.

Patient's Name _____ **J.M.** _____ Date of rating **2 – 26 – 70** _____

Rated by **H.G.** _____

<u>APHASIA SEVERITY RATING SCALE</u>

0. No usable speech or auditory comprehension.

(1.) All communication is through fragmentary expression; great need for inference, questioning and guessing by the listener. The range of information which can be exchanged is limited, and the listener carries the burden of communication.

2. Conversation about familiar subjects is possible with help from the listener. There are frequent failures to convey the idea, but patient shares the burden of communication with the examiner.

3. The patient can discuss <u>almost all everyday problems</u> with little or no assistance. However, reduction of speech and/or comprehension make conversation about certain material difficult or impossible.

4. Some obvious loss of fluency in speech or facility of comprehension, without significant limitation on ideas expressed or form of expression.

5. Minimal discernible speech handicaps; patient may have subjective difficulties which are not apparent to listener.

RATING SCALE PROFILE OF SPEECH CHARACTERISTICS

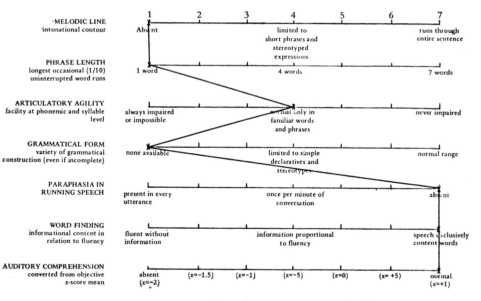

FIGURE 8.   Speech profile ratings of a Broca's aphasic.

commensurate with the patient's impaired fluency level. The parietal lobe cluster is at near-normal levels. A WAIS performance-scale I.Q. was 97, but when rescored without time limits, it was 127.

Examination of the speech characteristics profile again shows the typical Broca's aphasia pattern, with uniformly low speech melody, articulation and phrase-length, absence of paraphasia, and superiority of word-finding to the general fluency level. The auditory comprehension scale, based on the mean z-scores of the auditory comprehension cluster, is at the near-normal level.

Wernicke's Aphasia

(Head—"Syntactic Aphasia"; Goldstein—"Sensory Aphasia"; Luria—"Acoustic Aphasia"; Weisenburg and McBride—"Receptive Aphasia.")

This syndrome, the most common of the "fluent" aphasias, usually depends on a lesion in the posterior portion of the first temporal gyrus of the left hemisphere. The critical features of this syndrome are impaired auditory comprehension and fluently articulated, but paraphasic speech. The impairment of auditory comprehension is evident even at the one-word level. The patient may repeat the examiner's words uncomprehendingly, or with paraphasic distortions. At severe levels, auditory comprehension may be zero, while paraphasia is so pervasive as to produce meaningless jargon. Paraphasia may include both sound transpositions (literal paraphasia) and word substitutions (verbal paraphasia). In addition, word-finding difficulty is an almost constant feature of this disorder, while reading and writing are usually severely impaired as well.

Though the grammar of these patients is often incorrect, there is usually free use of complex verb tenses, embedded subordinate clauses, and other departures from simple declarative word order. Their syntax is, therefore, described as "paragrammatic," rather than "agrammatic."

Repetition usually results in paraphasic distortion of the examiner's words, with the appearance of neologisms and irrelevant insertions. These patients often add a word or phrase or use a more complex form than that given—a feature termed "augmentation." Another frequent concomitant of this disorder is a press of speech, often at a rate greater than normal, while the patient is unaware of anything wrong with his speech.

A patient with Wernicke's aphasia may sound like a normal speaker from a distance, because of his fluency and the normal melodic contour of his speech. At milder levels, auditory comprehension difficulty is improved to the point where only complex statements are misunderstood. Paraphasia, too, may become only an occasional feature and the patient starts to demonstrate awareness of his own errors, by self-correction and inhibition. Because the posterior location of the lesion usually spares the motor area, these patients may continue to use the right hand for writing and, in many cases, they preserve their natural handwriting, although the content of their written production is unintelligible. Occasional Wernicke's aphasics produce fluent, but paraphasic writing which parallels their speech in its disorganized, rambling style, in which there is repetitive use of certain words or phrases and a dearth of substantives and concrete action words. The following is a sample of writing obtained from such a patient: "His wife saw the wonting to wofin to a house with the umblelor. Then he left the wonding then he too to the womin and to the umbella up stairs. His wife carry it upstairs. Then the house did not go faster thern and tell go in the without within pain where it is whire in the herce in stock."

The theoretical model proposed for this defect is that Wernicke's area is the crossroad for all meaningful associations to sound patterns and for performances (such as reading and writing) which have been learned in conjunction with the auditory component of words. Its location, adjacent to the primary cortical auditory center

(Heschl's gyrus), suggests that it plays the role of association area for audition, analogously with the other association areas, visual and motor, which are contiguous to the primary cortical end-stations for those modalities.

It is readily understandable that injury to such a center may reduce performances which depend on past and current auditory experience; however, one can only conjecture on the mechanism by which such injury may also produce paraphasia, excessively rapid speech and anomia, while leaving syntactic automatisms relatively intact. Wernicke and others have suggested that paraphasia is the result of defective auditory monitoring of the speech output. This explanation fits well with the patient's unawareness of errors, but does not explain where the inappropriate speech comes from in the first place. Pressure of speech and resistance to interruption sometimes strike the listener as a result of the patient's failure to experience the

"closure" which comes with the awareness of having finished expressing an idea. Depending on the patient's temperament and drive to express himself, he may press on blindly in speech, reaching for the elusive sense of having said what he intended.

CONFIGURATION OF TEST SCORES. The degree of severity of the Wernicke aphasic may fall at any level from "0" (no communication possible in either direction) to "4," the latter being patients who, after extended, virtually normal conversation, break into occasional paraphasic irrelevancies. Like the very mild Broca's aphasic, they cannot be distinguished reliably from mild anomics at severity levels "4" and "5," where diagnostic distinctions tend to break down.

Figure 9 shows, in its shaded area, the range of ratings consistent with Wernicke's aphasia.

The Aphasia Test z-score profiles show auditory comprehension and severity scores lower than fluency. Naming is also usually

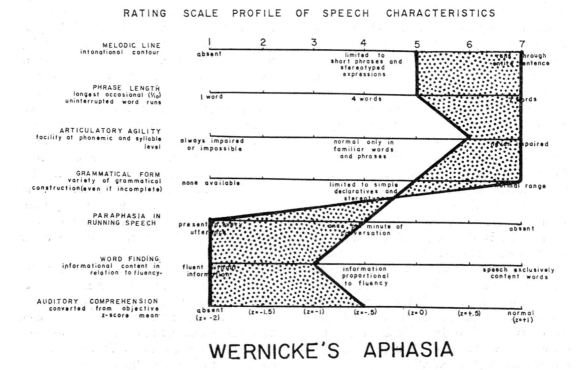

FIGURE 9.   Range of speech profile ratings characteristic of Wernicke's aphasia.

below the fluency level. All of the paraphasia indicators are elevated. Repetition
is commensurate with severity, and both
reading and writing clusters are depressed.

A CASE OF WERNICKE'S APHASIA. A.M., a
fifty-six-year-old physician, suffered a vascular accident diagnosed as a thrombosis in
the distribution of the left middle cerebral
artery, with effects extending posteriorly to
the angular gyrus. The episode occurred in
January, 1963, eight months prior to his
examination. By the time he was seen, his
initial right hemiparesis had cleared, leaving
only a mild hyperreflexia on the right, along
with a right homonymous hemianopia.
Sensation was normal. On examination by
Dr. Geschwind, A.M. was noted to present
the classical picture of Wernicke's aphasia,
with difficulty in all language input and
output modalities, but with fluent, easily
articulated paraphasic speech.

The following transcript of the "cookie
theft" narrative reveals the typical pattern
of compound and complex sentence structures, which get nowhere because semantically meaningless sequences are juxtaposed.
Paraphasia consists of totally irrelevant
English words, neologisms and repetitious
overuse of phrases built around the words,
"time" and "work."

"Well this is . . . mother is away here
working her work out o' here to get her
better, but when she's looking, the two boys
looking in the other part. One their small
tile into her time here. She's working
another time because she's getting, too. So
the two boys work together an one is sneakin'
around here, making his . . . work an' his
further funnas his time he had. He an' the
other fellow were running around the work
here, while mother another time she was
doing that without everything wrong here.
It isn't right, because she's making a time
here of work time here, letting mother
getting all wet here about something. The
kids aren't right here because they don't
just say one here and one here—that's all
right, although the fellow here is breakin'

between the two of them, they're comin'
around too."

Examination of the z-score profile for
A.M. reveals a severity rating of "1" and
aphasia subscores at or near the zero level
in all clusters representing purposeful use
of linguistic skills, e.g., auditory comprehension, naming, reading, repetition and
writing. Thus, he might be considered a
global aphasic from these scores alone, if
we did not also see a very high rating in
fluency and a large count of paraphasias in
extended utterances, which mark him as a
Wernicke's aphasic. It should be noted
that the opportunity for A.M. to produce
paraphasias during formal testing was much
reduced because the speech production tests
were all abridged in view of the irrelevancy
of his replies.

The scores on the subtests of the parietal
lobe battery are uniformly low, in accordance
with the clinical observations leading to the
inference of a Sylvian lesion extending
posteriorly towards the angular gyrus.

This profile of speech characteristics is a
classical one for Wernicke's aphasia with the
four upper-scale ratings at or near the normal
end and the three lower scales reflecting
ratings of maximum abnormality.

Anomia

(Head—"Nominal Aphasia"; Wepman—
"Semantic Aphasia"; Goldstein—"Amnesic
Aphasia.")

The syndromes of Wernicke's aphasia and
of anomia do not have a sharp boundary,
although the classic forms of each of these
"fluent" aphasias are unmistakably distinct.
Not only are there cases at every point
along the continuum of symptoms between
these two syndromes, but some patients,
who appear initially as full-blown Wernicke
aphasics, evolve into typical anomics in the
course of their recovery.

The major feature of anomic aphasia is
the prominence of word-finding difficulty in
the context of fluent, grammatically well-
formed speech. It differs from Wernicke's

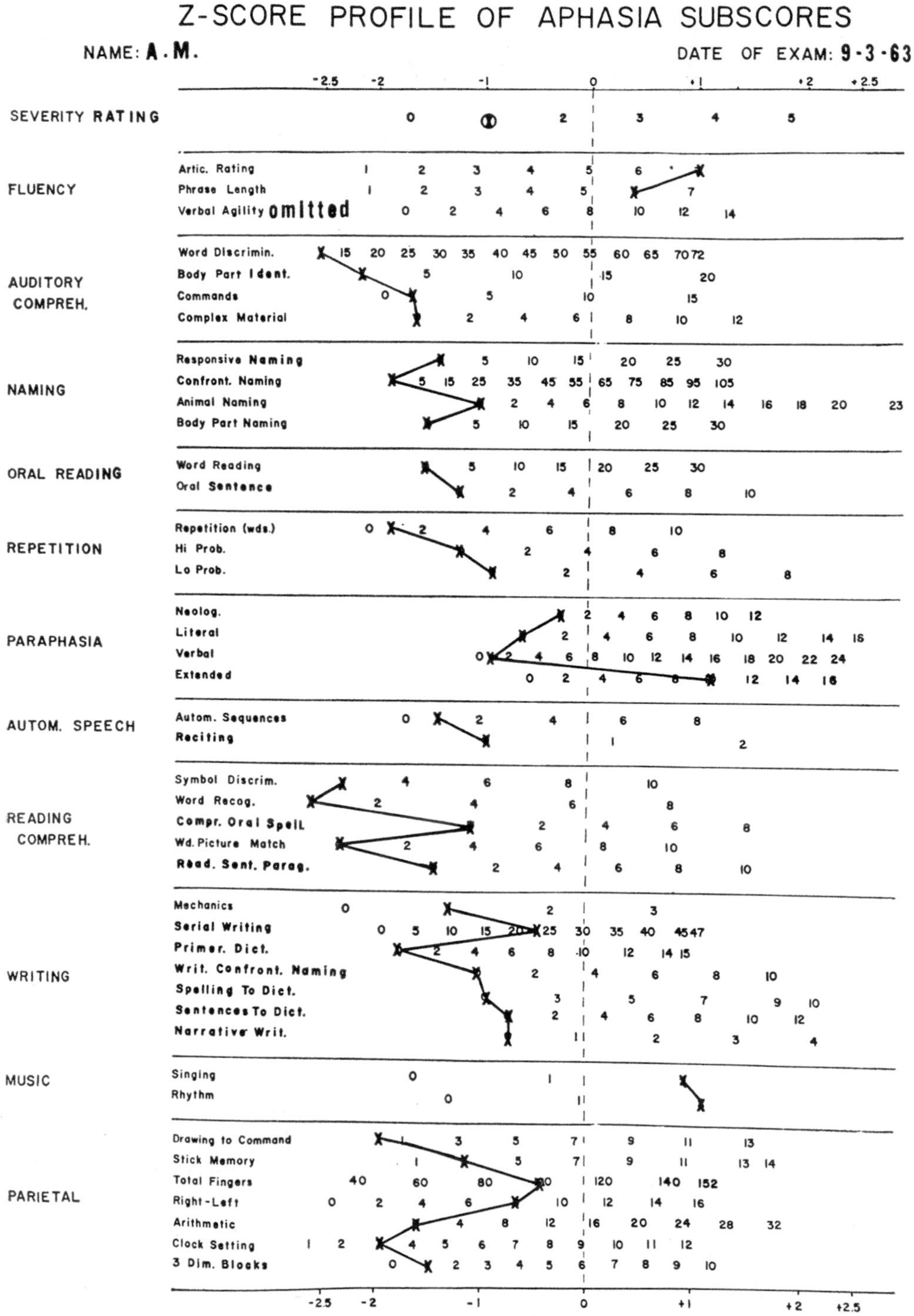

FIGURE 10.   Z-score profile of a Wernicke's aphasic.

Patient's Name **A.M.**   Date of rating **2-7-70**

Rated by **H.G.**

APHASIA SEVERITY RATING SCALE

0. No usable speech or auditory comprehension.

(1.) All communication is through fragmentary expression; great need for inference, questioning and guessing by the listener. The range of information which can be exchanged is limited, and the listener carries the burden of communication.

2. Conversation about familiar subjects is possible with help from the listener. There are frequent failures to convey the idea, but patient shares the burden of communication with the examiner.

3. The patient can discuss <u>almost all everyday problems</u> with little or no assistance. However, reduction of speech and/or comprehension make conversation about certain material difficult or impossible.

4. Some obvious loss of fluency in speech or facility of comprehension, without significant limitation on ideas expressed or form of expression.

5. Minimal discernible speech handicaps; patient may have subjective difficulties which are not apparent to listener.

RATING SCALE PROFILE OF SPEECH CHARACTERISTICS

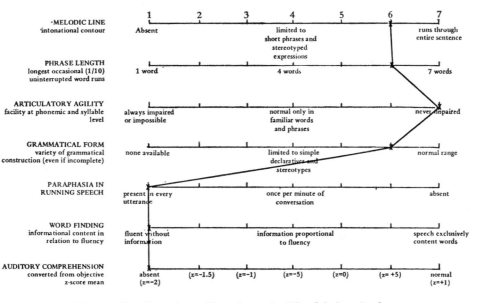

FIGURE 11. Speech profile ratings of a Wernicke's aphasic.

aphasia in the absence of literal and verbal paraphasia, and in the relative intactness of auditory comprehension. The classical anomic aphasic speaks freely, but with a dramatic emptiness of substantive words in his speech. In free conversation, some anomic aphasics are extremely facile in producing circumlocutions for their missing words. These circumlocutions may sound bizarre because of their vagueness, e.g., for "I had an operation on my head," one may hear, "I had one of them up there," or, with more specific circumlocutory terms, "I had a thing done up where your hair is." Testing of object-naming to confrontation will produce dramatic failures in extreme cases. Often, however, a patient whose conversation is strikingly empty of content names most objects quite promptly and a naming deficit is brought out only by pressing for less common words and for names of parts of objects (e.g., "point" of pencil, "teeth" of comb, "band" of watch).

While auditory comprehension is relatively good, the patient sometimes fails to recognize or accept a proffered word which he has been unable to evoke himself. For example, shown a wallet, the patient may say, "That's a purse." When asked if "wallet" would not be a better term, he may reject it, say it makes no difference which word is used or say, evasively, "You can call it that if you like." A recent study (Goodglass, Gleason and Hyde, 1970) reveals that these patients have significantly poorer comprehension of isolated nouns and verbs, with respect to their overall comprehension level, than do other types of patients.

Reading and writing may vary over a wide range from patient to patient. Anomia is often based on a temporal-parietal injury which may extend into the angular gyrus, which is most sensitive for disturbances of written language. In these cases, severe alexia and agraphia are part of the picture. Other patients, however, read at a functional level and write as they speak. Occasionally, a patient of this type will spell orally or

write a word which he cannot produce, suggesting that the spelled version of the word is learned and stored in parallel with the auditory model, but independently of it. Close examination of these cases shows that these acts of spelling are sporadic and that the writing of object-names is not much better than the verbalization. In spite of its frequent association with angular gyrus lesions, anomia is the least reliably localizable of the aphasic syndromes. It is commonly the first language disturbance with growing brain tumors which may exert pressure, though remote from the recognized language areas.

CONFIGURATION OF TEST SCORES. Anomic aphasics of severe degree are quite rare, and the severity rating of a patient of this type is usually "3" or "4." The speech profile of the classical form of this disorder is distinguished from a normal profile only by the word-finding scale, which is displaced towards the extreme of "fluent without information." The range of ratings consistent with anomic aphasia is included in the shaded area of Figure 12.

The Aphasia Test z-score profiles show both the fluency and auditory comprehension scores higher than the severity rating, although all are likely to be above the midpoint of the scales. Visual Confrontation Naming is lower than the foregoing scores, but only in extreme cases does it fall below the mean of "0." Paraphasia scores are low, except for "other" or "extended" paraphasia (last column) which may reflect occurrences of circumlocution during the test. Repetition is high, while reading and writing scores are unpredictable.

A CASE OF ANOMIC APHASIA. R. D. was a fifty-four-year-old, right-handed man who, though he had only eight years of formal schooling, had worked as a ship designer and had written a small book on ship design. He had suffered the onset of a right hemiplegia and speech difficulty without unconsciousness three months prior to his admission to the aphasia unit. By the time of his

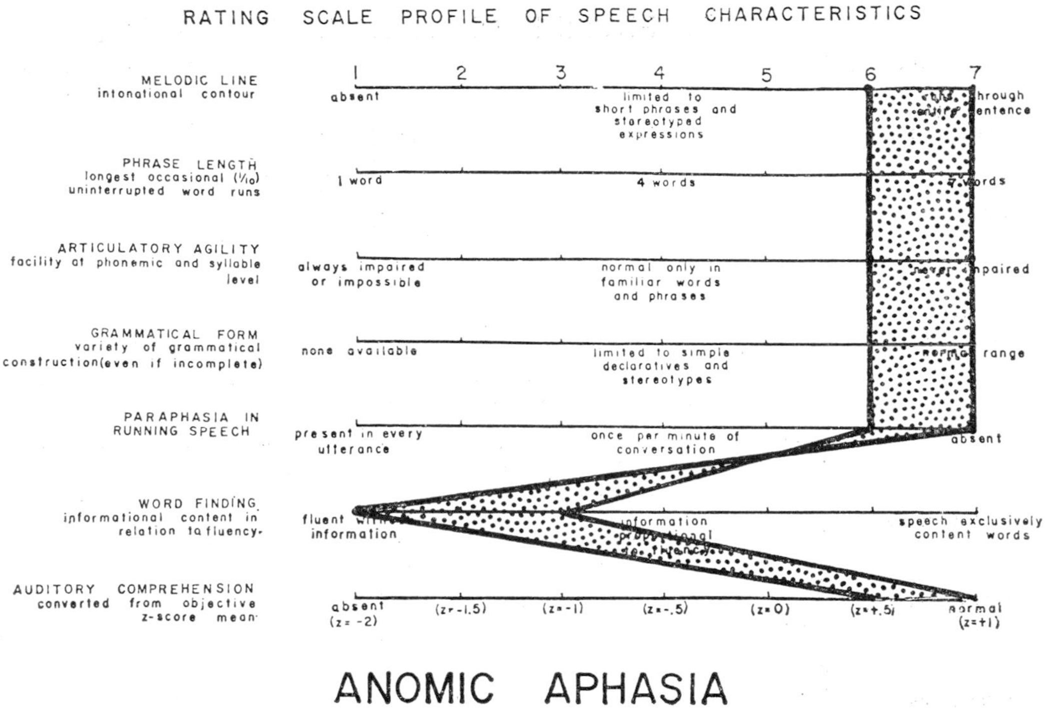

RATING SCALE PROFILE OF SPEECH CHARACTERISTICS

ANOMIC APHASIA

FIGURE 12. Range of speech profile ratings characteristic of anomic aphasia.

admission, his motor status had improved, with only residual weakness of his right arm. There was cortical sensory loss in the right arm only. Arteriogram revealed a complete occlusion of the left middle cerebral artery, but radioactive brain scan revealed a lesion confined to the left parieto-occipital region.

The neurologist's examination found his spontaneous speech clear, fluent and in full sentences, but reduced in rate and showing obvious word-finding difficulty. He was described as severely alexic and agraphic, having right-left confusion and apraxia for facial movements.

An example of his capacity for sentence organization from his free conversation is the following response to a question about the onset of his illness. "For three days, it was just a little bit here, then, all of a sudden, it just spread all over."

The sentences in his "cookie theft" narrative are grammatically somewhat simpler, being strung together by "and" connections.

This narrative shows most strikingly the word-finding difficulty and the substitution of indefinites for nouns which he cannot evoke:

"This is a boy and that's a boy an' that's a . . . thing! (Laughs.) An' this is goin' off pretty soon (points to toppling stool). This is a . . . a place that this is mostly in (Examiner: "Could you name the room . . . a bathroom?") No . . . kitchen . . . kitchen. An' this is a girl . . . an' that something that they're running an' they've got the water going down here . . ."

The patient received a severity rating of "2," indicating that conversation about familiar subjects is possible with help from the listener. Inspection of the z-score profile reveals that fluency is high and word-finding is low, a configuration consistent with any of the posterior aphasias. Looking at the auditory comprehension scales, we note that, in spite of failures in word discrimination and body-part comprehension, those

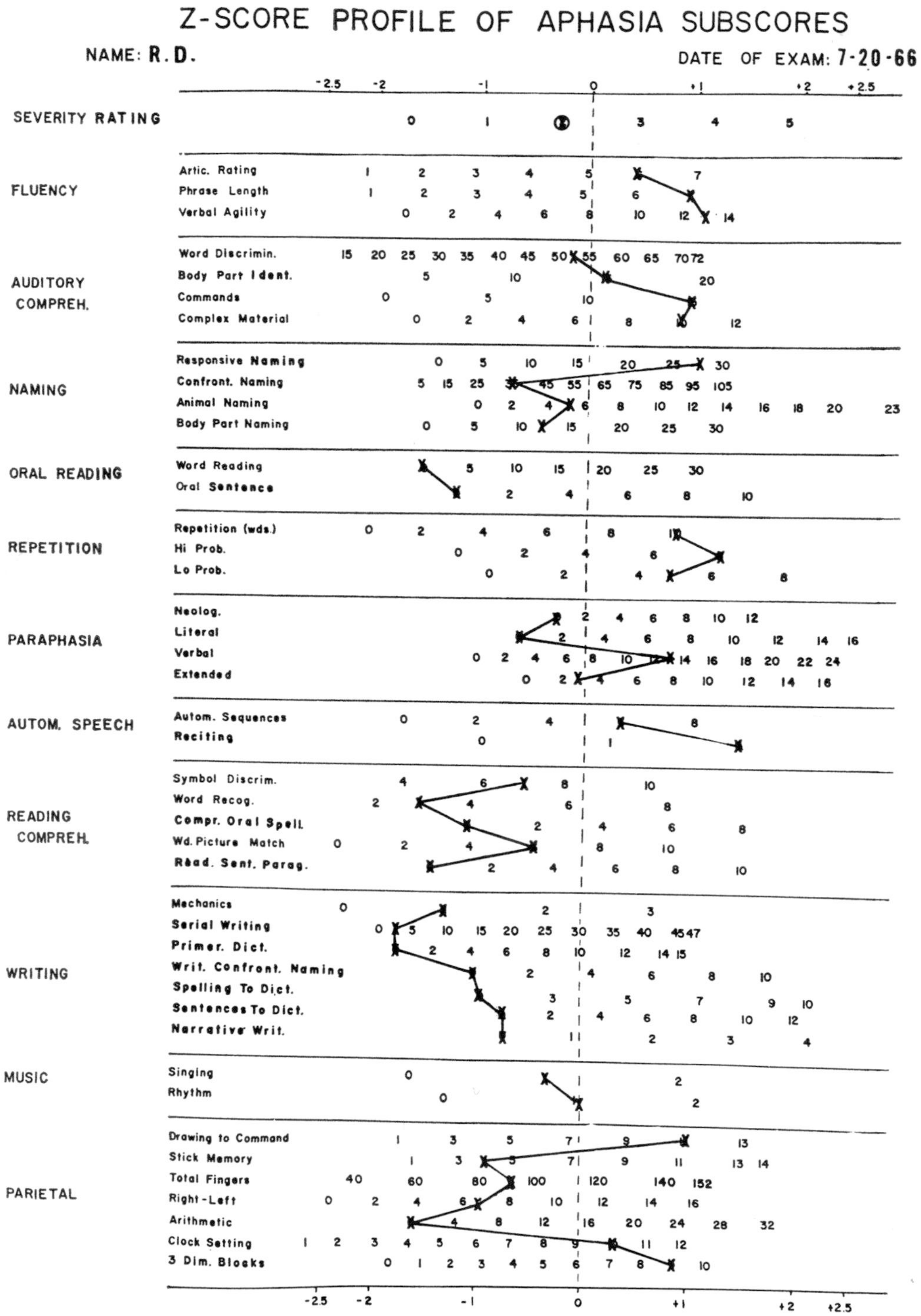

Z-SCORE PROFILE OF APHASIA SUBSCORES

NAME: **R.D.**   DATE OF EXAM: **7-20-66**

FIGURE 13.   Z-score profile of an anomic aphasic.

Patient's Name __R.D.__   Date of rating __2-26-70__
                                                     Rated by __H.G.__

<u>APHASIA SEVERITY RATING SCALE</u>

0. No usable speech or auditory comprehension.

1. All communication is through fragmentary expression; great need for inference,
    questioning and guessing by the listener. The range of information which can be
    exchanged is limited, and the listener carries the burden of communication.

②. Conversation about familiar subjects is possible with help from the listener. There are
    frequent failures to convey the idea, but patient shares the burden of communication
    with the examiner.

3. The patient can discuss <u>almost all everyday problems</u> with little or no assistance.
    However, reduction of speech and/or comprehension make conversation about certain
    material difficult or impossible.

4. Some obvious loss of fluency in speech or facility of comprehension, without significant
    limitation on ideas expressed or form of expression.

5. Minimal discernible speech handicaps; patient may have subjective difficulties which are
    not apparent to listener.

RATING SCALE PROFILE OF SPEECH CHARACTERISTICS

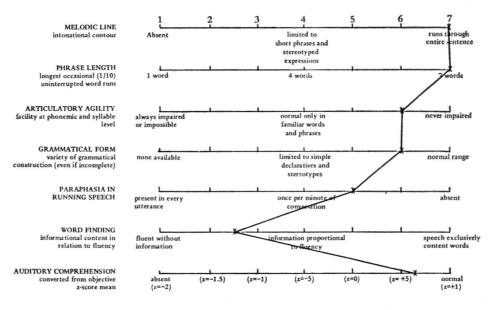

FIGURE 14.   Speech profile ratings of an anomic aphasic.

two scores lie slightly above the patient's general severity level, while the more complex comprehension scales are at near-normal levels. Severity of the aphasia seems chiefly due to the depressed naming scores, which (except for responsive naming) fall *lower* on the z-score scale than does the severity rating and certainly well below the comprehension rating. This makes anomic aphasia the best-fitting syndrome. Conduction aphasia is excluded by the high repetition cluster and the absence of literal paraphasias.

The subtest profile also reflects the severe impairment of written language noted by the neurologist. Both reading and writing clusters lie entirely below the oral language scores. This configuration is not a constant feature in anomic aphasia. It indicates a lesion implicating the posterior temporo-parietal region (angular gyrus) which is also reflected in poor finger localization, right-left confusion and acalculia on the "parietal lobe" battery.

Inspection of the Rating Scale Profile of Speech Characteristics shows some deviation from the classical profile of anomia, in that some minimal articulatory deficit and restriction in variety of grammatical form are noted. Verbal paraphasias occur somewhat more in this patient's speech than in classical forms of anomia, while the word-finding difficulty itself is less severe than is typically the case.

Conduction Aphasia

(Goldstein—"Central Aphasia"; Luria—"Afferent Motor Aphasia.")

This is the name applied to the syndrome in which repetition is disproportionately severely impaired in relation to the level of fluency in spontaneous speech and to the near normal level of auditory comprehension. While it is considered one of the "fluent" aphasias, the fluency may be restricted to brief bursts of speech. In these cases, the patients are unlike Broca's aphasics in that they usually produce well-articulated sequences of English phonemes with normal intonation and initiate a variety of syntactic patterns. The outstanding speech difficulty is in the proper choice and sequencing of their phonemes, so that *literal paraphasia* constantly interferes with production. Sometimes the patient's struggle with his literal paraphasia results in an output like that of a Broca's aphasic and it may be difficult to differentiate these two types of aphasia on the basis of the articulation rating scale. In the more fluent conduction aphasic, an *anomic* component is very prominent and the patient may run along fluently until he encounters a substantive or a principal verb, at which point he struggles paraphasically, with repeated approximations, to untangle the sounds of this word. This "zeroing in" behavior is referred to as "conduite d'approche" in the French literature. Unlike the Wernicke aphasic, the conduction aphasic is acutely aware of his inaccuracy and rejects his incorrect efforts.

It is primarily in repetition that we see literal paraphasic intrusions interfering with the intended output. While familiar single words and short, conversational expressions rarely present difficulty for repetition, the conduction aphasic is baffled by polysyllabic words, and the type of sentences included in the "low-probability" sentence repetitions of the aphasia test. Even here, however, self-correction often results in correct final output, so that the score is insensitive to this defect. Whereas the articulation of a Broca's aphasic is always aided by a model for repetition, the reverse is true for the conduction aphasic.

One of the striking phenomena in repetition difficulties is the difference between number-language and other speech. These patients often respond perfectly normally to the request for number repetition, in striking contrast to their groping attempts at other words. Moreover, errors with number repetition take the form of verbal paraphasia (word-substitution) rather than literal paraphasia. When numbers are combined with words (e.g., "84 divided by

7 equals 12"), the contrast between them may emerge dramatically. (See supplementary tests for repetition in Chapter 5.)

The auditory comprehension of these patients is often completely intact. They were found to have a normal mean score in auditory comprehension vocabulary—superior to that of anomics.

Conduction aphasia is attributed by some (e.g., Geschwind, 1965) to a lesion in the arcuate fasciculus—a fiber pathway believed to carry information from Wernicke's area to Broca's area. It is affected by a lesion deep to the supramarginal gyrus, which also commonly involves the sensory area for the upper right limb.

CONFIGURATION OF TEST SCORES. Conduction aphasics are not readily diagnosable at the most severe levels (0 or 1) since, if their speech is very sparse, they may resemble Broca's aphasics or, if they are more fluent, they may have some of the impaired comprehension and verbal and neologistic paraphasia of Wernicke aphasics. Unambiguous cases of this syndrome may range from severity level "2" to "4." Their profiles on the speech characteristics scale are variable at several points, notably for phrase length and articulation. Since the profile has no scale for repetition, this diagnosis cannot be made unambiguously from the profile.

Paraphasia in running speech may occur in some patients who do not bother to self-correct. Others will always stop at an error, interrupting their flow. The auditory comprehension scale is uniformly high.

On the z-score summary of the Diagnostic Aphasia Test, auditory comprehension is superior to severity and fluency levels. Repetition is depressed, especially the low-probability sentences. The paraphasia cluster shows an elevation in literal paraphasia and sometimes in neologistic paraphasia. Reading comprehension and writing scores are usually on a par with the severity rating.

A CASE OF CONDUCTION APHASIA. K.L. was a twenty-year-old male, high school graduate who, while at a U.S. Air Force base,

suffered a 22-caliber bullet wound in the head on January 16, 1964, two months prior to this examination. The bullet entered the left lower mid-parietal region and crossed the midline, coming to rest in the right parietal lobe. There were bilateral intracerebral hematomas and bone fragments in the path of the bullet. Bilateral craniotomy was performed to remove the bullet, drain and debride the wound.

When seen two months later, he had a very mild right-sided weakness, diminished position sense and increased two-point discrimination threshold in both hands with astereognosis bilaterally. His speech was described as fluent with good rhythm and occasional long sentences in free conversation. In repetition, however, he appeared dysarthric and spoke with effort. He was considered a conduction aphasic. His gunshot wound also was located precisely in a position to interfere with the path of the arcuate fasciculus, consistent with the anatomical rationale for conduction aphasia.

The following transcript of narrative description of the "cookie theft" picture is typical of his speech. It illustrates his capacity for extended grammatical runs of speech, his generally self-corrected word-finding slips and the phonemic substitutions which appear, principally in substantives, in a general context of facile articulation.

"Well this um . . . somebody's . . . ah mahther is takin the . . . washin' the dayshes an' the water . . . the water is falling . . . is flowing all over the place, an' the kids sneakin' out in back behind her, takin' the cookies in the . . . out of the top in the . . . what do you call that? (Examiner: "Shelf?") Yes . . . and there's a . . . then the girl . . . not the girl . . . the boy who's getting the cookies is on this ah . . . strool an' startin' to fall off. That's about all I see."

Inspection of the rating scale profile (Figure 16) reveals rating at or near the normal position of all scales except those for paraphasia and word-finding. His severity rating was "3." This, in conjunction with

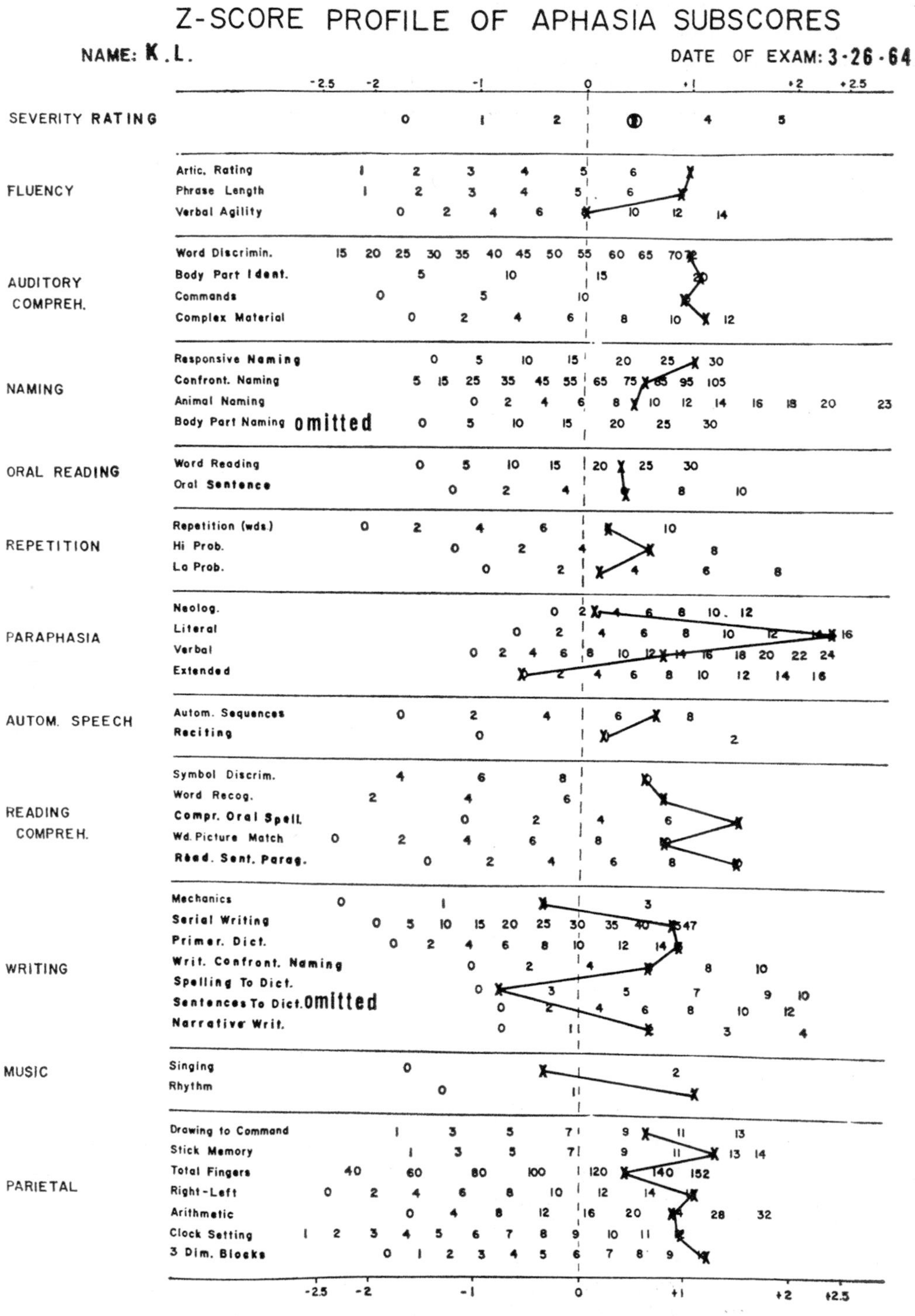

Z-SCORE PROFILE OF APHASIA SUBSCORES

NAME: K.L.   DATE OF EXAM: 3·26·64

-2.5 -2 -1 0 +1 +2 +2.5

SEVERITY RATING — 0 1 2 3 4 5

FLUENCY
- Artic. Rating — 1 2 3 4 5 6
- Phrase Length — 1 2 3 4 5 6
- Verbal Agility — 0 2 4 6 8 10 12 14

AUDITORY COMPREH.
- Word Discrimin. — 15 20 25 30 35 40 45 50 55 60 65 70
- Body Part Ident. — 5 10 15
- Commands — 0 5 10
- Complex Material — 0 2 4 6 8 10 12

NAMING
- Responsive Naming — 0 5 10 15 20 25 30
- Confront. Naming — 5 15 25 35 45 55 65 75 85 95 105
- Animal Naming — 0 2 4 6 8 10 12 14 16 18 20 23
- Body Part Naming omitted — 0 5 10 15 20 25 30

ORAL READING
- Word Reading — 0 5 10 15 20 25 30
- Oral Sentence — 0 2 4 8 10

REPETITION
- Repetition (wds.) — 0 2 4 6 8 10
- Hi Prob. — 0 2 4 8
- Lo Prob. — 0 2 4 8

PARAPHASIA
- Neolog. — 0 2 4 6 8 10 12
- Literal — 0 2 4 6 8 10 12 16
- Verbal — 0 2 4 6 8 10 12 14 16 18 20 22 24
- Extended — 2 4 6 8 10 12 14 16

AUTOM. SPEECH
- Autom. Sequences — 0 2 4 6 8
- Reciting — 0 2

READING COMPREH.
- Symbol Discrim. — 4 6 8
- Word Recog. — 2 4 6
- Compr. Oral Spell. — 0 2 4 6
- Wd. Picture Match — 0 2 4 6 8
- Read. Sent. Parag. — 0 2 4 6 8

WRITING
- Mechanics — 0 1 3
- Serial Writing — 0 5 10 15 20 25 30 35 40 47
- Primer. Dict. — 0 2 4 6 8 10 12 14
- Writ. Confront. Naming — 0 2 4 8 10
- Spelling To Dict. — 0 3 5 7 9 10
- Sentences To Dict. omitted — 0 2 4 6 8 10 12
- Narrative Writ. — 0 1 3 4

MUSIC
- Singing — 0 2
- Rhythm — 0 1

PARIETAL
- Drawing to Command — 1 3 5 7 9 11 13
- Stick Memory — 1 3 5 7 9 11 13 14
- Total Fingers — 40 60 80 100 120 140 152
- Right-Left — 0 2 4 6 8 10 12 14
- Arithmetic — 0 4 8 12 16 20 28 32
- Clock Setting — 1 2 3 4 5 6 7 8 9 10 11
- 3 Dim. Blocks — 0 1 2 3 4 5 6 7 8 9

-2.5 -2 -1 0 +1 +2 +2.5

FIGURE 15. Z-score profile of a conduction aphasic.

Patient's Name _____ **K . L .** _____ Date of rating ___ **2 – 26 – 70** _____

Rated by ___ **H.G.** _____

APHASIA SEVERITY RATING SCALE

0. No usable speech or auditory comprehension.

1. All communication is through fragmentary expression; great need for inference, questioning and guessing by the listener. The range of information which can be exchanged is limited, and the listener carries the burden of communication.

2. Conversation about familiar subjects is possible with help from the listener. There are frequent failures to convey the idea, but patient shares the burden of communication with the examiner.

③. The patient can discuss <u>almost all everyday problems</u> with little or no assistance. However, reduction of speech and/or comprehension make conversation about certain material difficult or impossible.

4. Some obvious loss of fluency in speech or facility of comprehension, without significant limitation on ideas expressed or form of expression.

5. Minimal discernible speech handicaps; patient may have subjective difficulties which are not apparent to listener.

RATING SCALE PROFILE OF SPEECH CHARACTERISTICS

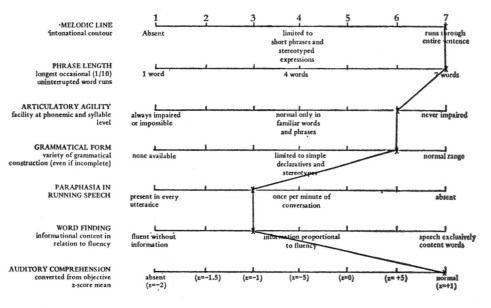

FIGURE 16.   Speech profile ratings of a conduction aphasic.

the normal auditory comprehension score, is typical for conduction aphasia. The z-score profile (Figure 15) shows that, while absolute scores for repetition are only moderately depressed, they are lower than the fluency and auditory comprehension levels. Moreover, the count of literal paraphasias is by far the highest in the paraphasia group. This patient performs at the top of our reading scale, but earns only a score of "1" in spelling from dictation. Nevertheless, he could write an incomplete but relevant sentence about the cookie theft, in which, through his poor spelling, omissions and partly illegible letters, a well-formulated sentence could be discerned.

The patient's scores on the spatial-somatognosic-quantitative subtests of the "Parietal Lobe Battery" are all within the normal range, reflecting the integrity of the posterior temporo-parietal functions in this circumscribed midparietal lesion.

Transcortical Sensory Aphasia

(Geschwind—"Isolated Speech Area" Syndrome.)

This syndrome, which is rather rare, is characterized by the remarkable preservation of repetition in the context of the features of a severe Wernicke's aphasia. The postulated pathophysiology of this syndrome (Geschwind, Segarra and Quadfasel, 1968) is that the auditory-vocal mechanism of the speech area, represented by the Wernicke-Broca area complex, is spared, but cut off from the rest of the brain by a band of infarcted brain tissue. Lesions of this type (referred to as "watershed" lesions) may be produced by vascular insufficiency. The rationale for the set of symptoms is that Wernicke's area can perform its operations of auditory analysis and classification, and pass its information along to an intact Broca's area to permit repetition. However, the isolation of this portion of the speech system prevents any interaction between the knowledge, intention and perceptions of the rest of the brain and those of the isolated speech mechanism.

The typical patient with this disorder does not initiate speech on his own. When addressed, he replies with well-articulated, but irrelevant paraphasia which may include both actual English words and neologisms. He is totally unable to name to confrontation but usually offers grossly irrelevant responses when so stimulated. These patients often echo the examiner's words instead of replying. However their ability to repeat is not limited to echoing, as they may, on request, listen to and repeat back correctly sentences of considerable length and complexity.

Along with the remarkable sparing of repetition, there is an unusual preservation of memorized material. Patients of this group may recite perfectly the Lord's Prayer or other familiar passages. They also sing, with the words, any songs that were known to them premorbidly, once given a start.

Written language is completely destroyed both for reading and writing.

APPEARANCE OF TEST PROFILE. The severity rating of a patient with transcortical sensory aphasia is most likely to be at level 1 or 2. The appearance of their Rating Scale Profile of Speech Characteristics differs in no way from that of Wernicke's aphasia, since their intact repetition is not reflected on this set of scales. The z-score profile sheet, however, will show all repetition scores elevated with respect to severity and auditory comprehension, with the remainder of the profile similar to that of Wernicke's aphasia.

A CASE OF TRANSCORTICAL SENSORY APHASIA. C.N. was a forty-nine-year-old male whose educational and occupational background were unknown. He had been injured in an automobile accident in August, 1963, sixteen months prior to his examination at the Boston VA Hospital. He had suffered a left temporo-parietal hematoma, which had been removed, and he had a plate over his skull defect. He had a severe hemiplegia.

On examination, he was socially appropriate and aware of his difficulty. His speech was described as normal in rate, rhythm, and length of phrases, but with an emptiness of relevant substantives, and runs of irrelevant jargon of English and neologistic words. He trailed off without completing the sense of his sentences. Auditory comprehension was moderately impaired, but would deteriorate during the course of a testing session. He was severely alexic and agraphic and completely apraxic. The words, "right" and "left," were devoid of meaning to him, although he could find his way easily about the hospital.

The striking feature of this patient was his remarkable ability to repeat long sentences, even foreign phrases, correctly in the face of his profound naming difficulty and paraphasia in other than repetition responses. He also had a strong urge to echo, which could be restrained only with repeated instructions.

Some examples of his confabulatory responses to naming of visual stimuli are:

for a cross: "Brazilian clothesbag"
for a thumb: "Argentine rifle"
for a metal ashtray: "beer-can thing"
for a necktie: "toenail . . . rusty nail"

Other examples of his jargon in extended utterances are, "He looks like he's up live walk . . . He looks like he's doing jack ofinarys . . . He lying wheaty . . . I don't know what you call that . . . He's taking souls."

The patient earned a severity rating of "1," as limited communication was possible through his partial comprehension of the examiner. (See Figure 18.) Inspection of the aphasia z-score profile (Figure 17) reveals high fluency in relation to his severity rating, placing him unambiguously among the posterior aphasics. The rest of the profile shows elevated repetition, automatic speech and paraphasia clusters in a context of minimal performance on all tests of propositional language, both oral and written. The tally of neologistic paraphasia, even though elevated, does not reflect his high propensity

for these utterances, because the subtests were discontinued after his early failures, reducing the opportunity for paraphasias. His scores on the parietal lobe battery are a series of total failures.

Inspection of the Profile of Speech Characteristics shows a configuration indistinguishable from that of a classical Wernicke aphasia. Only the high repetition and recitation scores on the aphasia battery reveal that this case is in the transcortical group. This is a case which illustrates the critical importance of repetition tests, and their evaluation in comparison to the level of other performances.

Transcortical Motor Aphasia

(Luria—"Dynamic Aphasia.")

As in the preceding syndrome, the term, "transcortical," implies that repetition is particularly intact in a setting of otherwise limited speech. This syndrome is marked by an absence of spontaneous speech, with some recovery of the ability to make brief replies to questions and fairly good confrontation naming ability. The patient has difficulty in initiating and organizing his response but, once initiated, it is usually well articulated. Auditory comprehension is relatively well spared, as are reading comprehension and oral reading. Repetition is remarkable in that it is prompt, well articulated, grammatically intact and free of difficulty of initiation which marks all other speech.

Alexia with Agraphia

Patients with a lesion in the posterior margin of the language area, i.e., the angular gyrus which bridges the posterior temporal and parietal regions, regularly present a defect in reading and writing, whereas speech and comprehension may be completely exempt from impairment.

In severe cases, the disturbance of reading may be so profound that the patient cannot match letters or words across styles of writing (upper to lower case, etc.), as tested

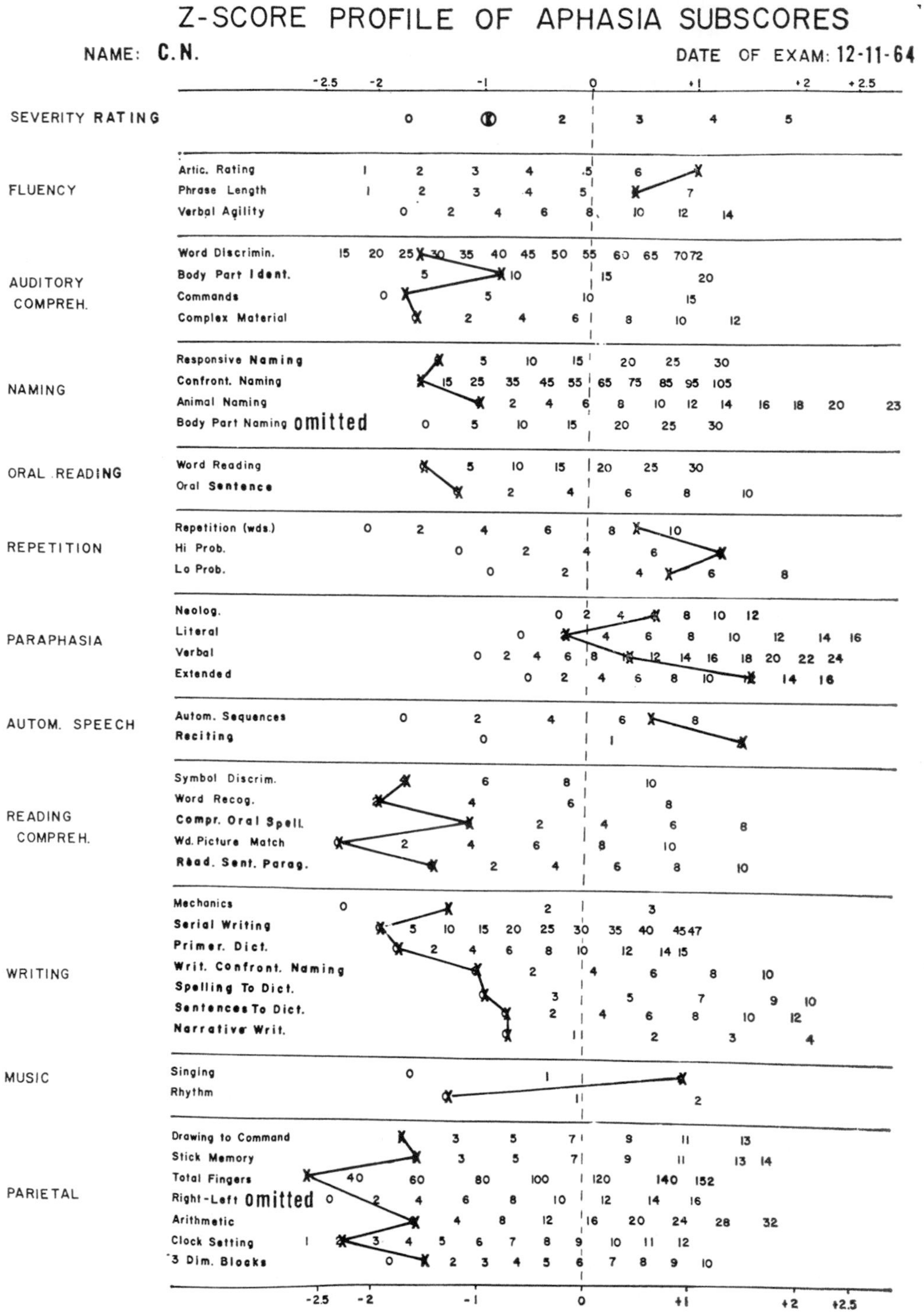

FIGURE 17.   Z-score profile of a transcortical sensory aphasic.

Patient's Name ___C.N._____ Date of rating __2-26-70___

Rated by __H.G._____

APHASIA SEVERITY RATING SCALE

0.   No usable speech or auditory comprehension.

(1.)   All communication is through fragmentary expression; great need for inference, questioning and guessing by the listener. The range of information which can be exchanged is limited, and the listener carries the burden of communication.

2.   Conversation about familiar subjects is possible with help from the listener. There are frequent failures to convey the idea, but patient shares the burden of communication with the examiner.

3.   The patient can discuss almost all everyday problems with little or no assistance. However, reduction of speech and/or comprehension make conversation about certain material difficult or impossible.

4.   Some obvious loss of fluency in speech or facility of comprehension, without significant limitation on ideas expressed or form of expression.

5.   Minimal discernible speech handicaps; patient may have subjective difficulties which are not apparent to listener.

RATING SCALE PROFILE OF SPEECH CHARACTERISTICS

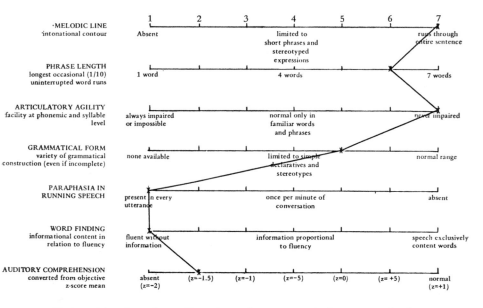

FIGURE 18.   Speech profile ratings of a transcortical sensory aphasic.

by the Symbol and Word Discrimination subtest. More often, letter recognition is spared and the patient can perform inconstantly with three- to four-letter primer words.

Writing is also severely impaired in that patients are unable to write letters from dictation or to transcribe from print into longhand, although slavish copying is usually preserved.

This syndrome may also occur in milder form with slow reading, spotted with misperceptions and failures to recognize even common words. In mild cases, elementary writing is preserved but gross errors in spelling are common. In the effort of writing, the patient loses track of the grammatical features and omits or misuses small words and inflectional endings, even though his oral speech is normal.

The anatomical localization of this syndrome in the angular gyrus usually brings along additional difficulties associated with this area. If speech is at all affected, the symptoms are those of a mild anomic aphasia. However, the complex of nonlanguage parietal lobe signs is most reliably present to some degree. These include a marked difficulty in calculation, including clock-setting, finger identification and right-left discrimination. The involvement of drawing and other visuo-spatial constructions is variable and may be quite severe. (For examination procedures in the associated nonverbal defects, refer to Chapter 6.)

CONFIGURATION OF TEST SCORES. Since the patient with alexia and agraphia may have normal oral language, his Rating Scale Profile may be indistinguishable from normal. However, the z-score summary sheet will show extremely low scores in the reading and writing clusters, and impairment in the parietal lobe group.

PURE APHASIAS

The "pure" aphasias have in common the feature of affecting only a single input or output modality, while leaving language virtually intact in all associated modalities.

Pure aphasias are quite rare, especially pure agraphia.

Aphemia

This disorder, which is also termed "subcortical motor aphasia," is an isolated disorder of articulation in which auditory comprehension, reading and writing are intact. At first, the patient may be unable to produce any speech sounds, even in isolation, either in imitation or spontaneously, failing automatic recitation, unlike Broca's aphasics. At this stage, the patient is truly anarthric, although he can phonate. The inability to imitate speech-like movements may or may not be paralleled by an apraxia for nonspeech oral movements.

As recovery takes place, articulation is painfully slow and awkward, but it is evident from the start that the patient speaks in grammatically complete sentences and has no word-finding difficulty.

Moreover, unlike the Broca's aphasic, whose articulation is facilitated by imitation, by the familiarity or by the automatic character of the utterance, the aphemic continues to show only a minimal relation between his articulatory difficulty and the linguistic nature of the speech content.

The supposed subcortical site to which the lesion is attributed makes logical sense in that it interrupts the final outflow of information from Broca's area to the speech effector system, without hampering cortical language activity.

Pure Word-deafness

Almost as rare as pure agraphia is a condition in which auditory comprehension of language is lost without affecting speech output, reading or writing. Patients with pure word-deafness (also referred to as "subcortical sensory aphasia") react to sounds, but their response, when addressed, is similar to that of a deaf person. Unlike the Wernicke aphasic, they do not recognize speech as consisting of familiar acoustic patterns and are thus generally unable to repeat what they hear. Fragments of the message which do get through are in the form of sound elements, so that partial success in repeating is always a phonetic approximation, never a paraphasic association, as in Wernicke's aphasia.

On those occasions when a word is perceived and repeated, the patient at once understands it, demonstrating that, again unlike the case of Wernicke's aphasia, there is no dissociation of meaning from the acoustic pattern of the word.

While pure forms of this disorder are rare indeed, it is more often found with some of the features of Wernicke's aphasia, e.g., occasional paraphasic responses.

The basic lesion for this disorder is one which destroys both the major primary auditory cortex (Heschl's gyrus) and the subcortical fibers, bringing information from the auditory association area of the minor hemisphere. Thus, in spite of a nearly intact Wernicke's area on the left, comprehension of speech is absent because no auditory input reaches this system, the adjacent auditory center being destroyed and the contralateral one isolated by interruption of transcallosal fibers. Wernicke's area continues to play its role in the production of speech and in reading and writing.

Pure Alexia (Pure Word-blindness)

The least rare of the pure aphasias is alexia without agraphia—a most paradoxical disorder in which the patient can write normally but cannot read even his own handwriting. While a description of this disorder dating to 1588 is cited by Benton (1964), it was Déjerine (1892) who first provided both the physiological rationale and the neuropathological verification of the mechanism for this syndrome.

The patient with pure alexia is ordinarily blind in the right visual field of each eye, but has no visual perceptual problems in his normal field. His speech is normal, including the ability to name objects visually presented. Not only does he fail to read

words, but even letters may be difficult or impossible; however, his comprehension of oral spelling is perfectly normal. By this means, he may use his limited ability to recognize individual letters to spell written words to himself and so achieve a laborious "reading." Number recognition is usually exempt from defect. Roman numerals, in spite of the fact that they are written with letters, are as well retained as arabic numbers.

A number of examiners of these patients report that they have an extraordinary difficulty in both naming and identifying colors from their spoken names, although they match and sort colors perfectly (Geschwind and Fusillo, 1966).

The usual lesion for this disorder is one which destroys the visual cortex of the left hemisphere and damages the splenium of the corpus callosum, the latter structure being essential for the communication between the two visual association areas. Thus, while the language area of the left hemisphere is undamaged, it is isolated from visual input. The ability to name objects may be spared because objects, unlike letters, arouse rich, multimodal sensory associations which are carried to the major hemisphere through other than the interrupted visual association pathways. In rare instances, visual object-naming is also affected, as well as reading, resulting in "optic aphasia" (Freund, 1889).

Pure Agraphia

The angular-gyrus-injured patient may suffer from a severe disorder of writing and spelling with only minimal involvement of reading. In these instances, as we have noted, other, nonverbal components of the angular gyrus syndrome are to be expected. A much rarer form of pure agraphia has been reported, attributed by Exner (1881) to a lesion of the foot of the second frontal convolution. This area lies in the motor association area and may represent a way station for the recoding of the output of Broca's area and/or the angular gyrus association areas into the form in which it can activate the effectors for writing movements. The rarity of pure agraphia is certainly due at least in part to the low probability of an isolated vascular lesion of the foot of the second frontal convolution. In addition, individual variation in the organization of the writing system may make only a few people susceptible to this disorder from a frontal lesion.

CALLOSAL DISCONNECTION SYNDROMES

The partial isolation of the two hemispheres through injury or surgical section of the corpus callosum results in aphasic-like behavior related to the minor side of the body (i.e., the left side, in right-handed patients).

Unilateral Tactile Aphasia

Tactile naming, on palpation of familiar objects with the eyes shut is normally as easy with either hand as to visual confrontation. Patients suffering from an interruption of callosal fibers may show a severe naming disorder only when palpating objects in the left hand, naming them promptly when the objects are transferred to the right hand. This unilateral anomia is not caused by lack of tactile recognition, because the patient can select from a multiple-choice array the object which he could not name, provided that the selection is performed with the left hand. He can draw the object with his left hand if it is not too complex (e.g., case of Geschwind and Kaplan, 1962).

Thus, while he "knows" what he has felt, this knowledge is confined to the non-speaking right cerebral hemisphere. The right hand cannot draw nor select by touch what the left hand has felt.

Unilateral Agraphia and Apraxia

On the expressive side, disconnection of the callosal pathways makes it impossible for the patient to write sensibly with the left hand, although he continues to do so normally with the right. Similarly, the callosal patient is unable to execute verbal commands involving the left limbs, whereas limb praxis to verbal command is intact on the right.

Hemi-optic Aphasia

When there has been a complete transection of the corpus callosum, extending to its posterior portion (splenium), objects experienced in the left visual field cannot be named, since no sensory information concerning them can reach the major hemisphere language area. Again, they can be picked out from multiple choice with the left hand, guided by the knowledge confined to the right side of the brain. This examination must ordinarily be conducted with a tachistoscopic arrangement in which the stimulus is flashed briefly to one side of the visual field to preclude scanning with both visual fields. No naturally occurring case of damage to both the splenium and anterior portions of the corpus callosum has been reported in which both visual fields were spared. Hemi-optic aphasia has been described only in cases of surgical intervention for the control of bilaterally spreading epileptic discharges (Gazzaniga and Sperry, 1967).

REFERENCES

Benton, A., "Contributions to aphasia before Broca." *Cortex*, 1964, *1*, 314–329.

Broca, P., "Perte de la parole. Ramollissement chronique et destruction partielle du lobe antérieur gauche du cerveau." *Bulletin de la Société d'anthropologie*, 1861, II, 235–238.

Critchley, M., *The Parietal Lobes*. New York, Hafner Publishing Company, 1966.

Déjerine, J., "Des différentes variétés de cécité verbale." *Memoires de la Société Biologique*, 1892, Fév. 27, 1–30. Abstract in *Brain*, 1893, *16*, 318–320.

Eisenson, J., *Examining for Aphasia*. New York, The Psychological Corporation, 1954.

Exner, S., *Lokalisation des Funktion der Grosshirnrinde des Menschen*. Wien, Braunmuller, 1881.

Freund, C. S., Uber optische aphasie und seelenblindheit. *Archiv. Psychiatrie Nervenkr.*, 1889, *20*, 276–297; 371–416.

Gazzaniga, M., and Sperry, R. W., "Language after section of the cerebral commissures." *Brain*, 1967, *90*, 131–148.

Geschwind, N., "Disconnexion syndromes in animals and man." *Brain*, 1965, *88*, 237–294, 585–644.

———, "Carl Wernicke, the Breslau School and the history of aphasia." In E. C. Carterette, ed., *Brain function, III, Speech, Language and Communication*, U.C.L.A. Forum in the Medical Sciences, No. 4, University of California Press, pp. 1–16, 1966.

——— and Fusillo, M., "Color naming defects in association with alexia." *Archives of Neurology*, 1966, *15*, 137–146.

——— and Kaplan, E., "A human cerebral deconnection syndrome." *Neurology*, 1962, *12*, 675, 685.

———, Segarra, J., and Quadfasel, F. A., "Isolation of the speech area." *Neuropsychologia*, 1968, *7*, 327–340.

Goldstein, K., *Language and Language Disturbance*. New York, Grune and Stratton, 1948.

——— and Scheerer, M., *Abstract and Concrete Behavior*. Psychological Monographs, *53*, 329, 1941.

Goodglass, H., Barton, M., and Kaplan, E., "Sensory modality and object-naming in aphasia." *Journal of Speech and Hearing Research*, 1968, *11*, 488–496.

———, Gleason, J., and Hyde, M., "Some dimensions of auditory language comprehension in aphasia." *Journal of Speech and Hearing Research*, 1970, *13*, 595–606.

——— and Kaplan, E., "Disturbance of gesture and pantomime in aphasia." *Brain*, 1963, *86*, 703–720.

———, Klein, H., Carey, P., and Jones, K. J., "Specific semantic word categories in aphasia." *Cortex*, 1966, *2*, 74–89.

———, Quadfasel, F. A., and Timberlake, W. H., "Phrase length and the type and severity of aphasia." *Cortex*, 1964, *1*, 133–153.

Head, H., *Aphasia and Kindred Disorders of Speech*. New York, Macmillan, 1926.

Hécaen, H., and Dubois, J., *Histoire de la Neuropsychologie du Langage*. Paris, Flammarion, 1969.

Kaplan, E., *Gestural Representation of Implement Usage: An Organismic Developmental Study*. Doctoral dissertation, Clark University, 1968.

Lichtheim, L., As cited in S. Freud, *On Aphasia*. New York, Universities Press, 1953.

Luria, A. R., *Higher Cortical Functions in Man*. New York, Basic Books, 1966.

——— "Factors and forms of aphasia." In A. V. S. de Reuck and M. O'Connor, eds., *Disorders of communication*. Boston, Little, Brown, 1964.

MacKay, D. G., "Phonetic factors in the perception and recall of spelling errors." *Neuropsychologia*, 1968, *6*, 321–325.

McCarthy, J., and Kirk, S. A., *Illinois Test of Psycholinguistic Abilities*. Urbana, University of Illinois, Institute of Research for Exceptional Children, 1966.

Schuell, H., *Differential Diagnosis of Aphasia with the Minnesota Test*. Minneapolis, University of Minnesota Press, 1965.

BOSTON DIAGNOSTIC APHASIA EXAMINATION

Date:

Patient: Case #:

Residence:

Age: Birthplace:

Date of birth:

Education: Grade completed:

                                                  At what age?:

Occupational history:

Language background (circle one):   *English only*   *Bilingual*
   (If bilingual, brief language history)

Handedness history (including data on other family members):

Nature and duration of present illness:

Localizing information:

Hemiplegia (circle one):   *Right*   *Left*   *Recovered*   *Absent*

Hemianopsia (circle one):   *Right*   *Left*   *Recovered*   *Absent*

EEG Focus:

Operative information:

Other localizing information (e.g., scan findings, arteriogram, etc.):

I. CONVERSATIONAL AND EXPOSITORY SPEECH

Conduct informal exchange, incorporating suggested questions, to elicit as many of the desired responses as possible. Record verbatim. Tape record, if possible.

a. Response to greeting. (Q. "HOW ARE YOU TODAY?" or equivalent):

b. Response with "yes" or "no." (Q. "HAVE YOU EVER BEEN IN THIS HOSPITAL BEFORE?" or "HAVE I TESTED YOU BEFORE?"):

c. Response with "I think so," or equivalent. (Q. "DO YOU THINK WE CAN HELP YOU?" or ". . . HAVE HELPED YOU?"):

d. Response with "I don't know" or equivalent. (Q. "WHEN ARE YOUR TREATMENTS GOING TO BE FINISHED?"):

e. Response with "I hope so" or equivalent. (Q. "BEFORE TOO LONG LET'S HOPE. WHAT DO YOU SAY?"):

f. "What is your full name?":

g. "What is your full address?" (Accept as correct any response which includes street and number or street and city.):

h. *Open-ended conversation:* In order to elicit as much free conversation as possible, it is suggested that examiner start with familiar topics such as, "What kind of work were you doing before you became ill?" and, "Tell me what happened to bring you to the hospital." Encourage patient to speak for at least *ten minutes*,

(4)

if possible. (Minimize use of "yes"-"no" questions and probing for specific facts.) If tape recording is not used, record as much as possible verbatim.

i. Presentation of picture. Show the test picture and tell patient to, "Tell everything you see going on in this picture." Point to neglected features of the picture and ask for elaboration if patient's response is skimpier than his apparent potential. A minute is usually enough time.

Cookie Theft (Card 1)

Patient's Name _____ Date of rating _____

Rated by _____

APHASIA SEVERITY RATING SCALE

0. No usable speech or auditory comprehension.

1. All communication is through fragmentary expression; great need for inference, questioning and guessing by the listener. The range of information which can be exchanged is limited, and the listener carries the burden of communication.

2. Conversation about familiar subjects is possible with help from the listener. There are frequent failures to convey the idea, but patient shares the burden of communication with the examiner.

3. The patient can discuss almost all everyday problems with little or no assistance. However, reduction of speech and/or comprehension make conversation about certain material difficult or impossible.

4. Some obvious loss of fluency in speech or facility of comprehension, without significant limitation on ideas expressed or form of expression.

5. Minimal discernible speech handicaps; patient may have subjective difficulties which are not apparent to listener.

RATING SCALE PROFILE OF SPEECH CHARACTERISTICS

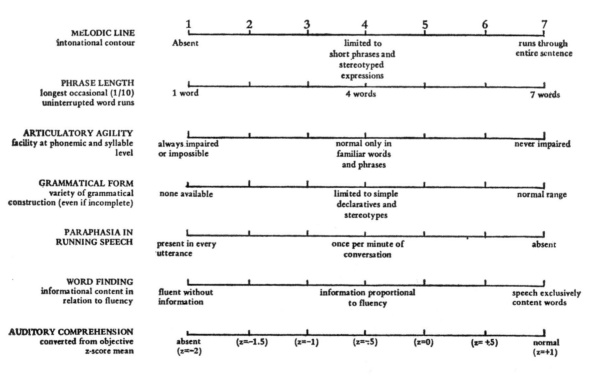

(6)

Z-SCORE PROFILE OF APHASIA SUBSCORES

NAME: DATE OF EXAM:

	-2.5	-2	-1	0	+1	+2	+2.5

SEVERITY RATING
0   1   2 | 3   4   5

FLUENCY

Artic. Rating	1 2 3 4 5	6 7
Phrase Length	1 2 3 4 5	6 7
Verbal Agility	0 2 4 6 8	10 12 14

AUDITORY COMPREH.

Word Discrimin.	15 20 25 30 35 40 45 50 55	60 65 70 72
Body Part Ident.	5 10	15 20
Commands	0 5 10	15
Complex Material	0 2 4 6	8 10 12

NAMING

Responsive Naming	0 5 10 15	20 25 30
Confront. Naming	5 15 25 35 45 55	65 75 85 95 105
Animal Naming	0 2 4 6	8 10 12 14 16 18 20 23
Body Part Naming	0 5 10 15	20 25 30

ORAL READING

| Word Reading | 0   5   10   15 | 20   25   30 |
| Oral Sentence | 0   2   4 | 6   8   10 |

REPETITION

Repetition (wds.)	0 2 4 6	8 10
Hi Prob.	0 2 4	6 8
Lo Prob.	0 2	4 6 8

PARAPHASIA

Neolog.	0 2 4 6 8 10 12
Literal	0 2 4 6 8 10 12 14 16
Verbal	0 2 4 6 8 10 12 14 16 18 20 22 24
Extended	0 2 4 6 8 10 12 14 16

AUTOM. SPEECH

| Autom. Sequences | 0   2   4 | 6   8 |
| Reciting | 0 | 1   2 |

READING COMPREH.

Symbol Discrim.	4 6 8	10
Word Recog.	2 4 6	8
Compr. Oral Spell	0 2	4 6 8
Wd. Picture Match	0 2 4 6	8 10
Read. Sent. Parag.	0 2 4	6 8 10

WRITING

Mechanics	0 1 2	3
Serial Writing	0 5 10 15 20 25 30	35 40 45 47
Primer. Dict.	0 2 4 6 8 10	12 14 15
Writ. Confront. Naming	0 2	4 6 8 10
Spelling To Dict.	0 3	5 7 9 10
Sentences To Dict.	0 2	4 6 8 10 12
Narrative Writ.	0 1	2 3 4

MUSIC

| Singing | 0   1 | 2 |
| Rhythm | 0   1 | 2 |

PARIETAL

Drawing to Command	1 3 5 7	9 11 13
Stick Memory	1 3 5 7	9 11 13 14
Total Fingers	40 60 80 100	120 140 152
Right-Left	0 2 4 6 8 10	12 14 16
Arithmetic	0 4 8 12	16 20 24 28 32
Clock Setting	1 2 3 4 5 6 7 8 9	10 11 12
3 Dim. Blocks	0 1 2 3 4 5 6	7 8 9 10

	-2.5	-2	-1	0	+1	+2	+2.5

II. AUDITORY COMPREHENSION

A. *Word Discrimination*

Present test Cards 2 and 3 separately. Have patient look over all pictures on the card presented before starting. Then ask him to point out each picture or symbol by saying, "Show me the _____." Rotate at random from one category to another. One repetition is permitted, on request. If the patient does not find the correct category, then show him the category, to the exclusion of the others, and repeat the name of the item to be identified. (Score in the "cued" column.) Correct discrimination ("identification") is scored 2 points if within 5 seconds, 1 point otherwise. Attention to the correct category without correct discrimination is scored ½ point (check category).

Card 2	IDENTIFICATION		CATE-GORY 1/2 point	CUE 1/2 point	FAIL 0	Card 3	IDENTIFICATION		CATE-GORY 1/2 point	CUE 1/2 point	FAIL 0
OBJECTS:	Under 5 seconds 2 points	Over 5 seconds 1 point				ACTIONS:	Under 5 seconds 2 points	Over 5 seconds 1 point			
chair						smoking					
key						drinking					
glove						running					
feather						sleeping					
hammock						falling					
cactus						dripping					
LETTERS:						COLORS:					
L						blue					
H						brown					
R						red					
T						pink					
S						gray					
G						purple					
FORMS:						NUMBERS:					
circle						7					
spiral						42					
square						700					
triangle						1936					
cone						15					
star						7000					

Raw Score: 0 10 17 24 31 38 45 52 59 66 72

B. *Body-part Identification*

Ask patient to point to the following body parts. Record incorrect responses.

Scoring: Items in the first two columns are scored 1 point if recognized promptly (within approximately 5 seconds) and ½ point if identified correctly, but after hesitation. The third column is for right-left discrimination and receives a total of 2 points if all 8 are correct (the body part may be incorrect as long as right-left discrimination is made), 1 point if 6 or 7 items are correct, otherwise 0.

	BODY-PART IDENTIFICATION								RIGHT-LEFT DISCRIMINATION		
	Correct		Fail		Correct		Fail			Correct	Failed
	<5″	>5″			<5″	>5″					
	1 point	1/2 point			1 point	1/2 point					
ear				wrist				right ear			
nose				thumb				left shoulder			
shoulder				thigh				left knee			
knee				chin				right ankle			
eyelid				elbow				right wrist			
ankle				lips				left thumb			
chest				eyebrow				right elbow			
neck				cheek				left cheek			
middle finger				index finger				8 correct 6–7 correct	2 points 1 point	

Raw Score: 0   2   4   6   8   10   12   14   16   18   20

C. *Commands*

Have the patient carry out the following commands, giving credit for each underlined element which he carries out. One repetition is permitted on request, but command must always be repeated as a whole, not broken up.

1. Make a *fist.*
2. Point to the *ceiling,* then to the *floor.*
   (After lining up a pencil, watch and card, in that order, on the table before the patient.)
3. Put the *pencil on top of the card,* then *put it back.*
4. Put the *watch* on the *other side of the pencil* and *turn over* the *card.*
5. Tap *each shoulder twice* with *two fingers* keeping your *eyes shut.*

Raw Score: 0   1   3   5   7   9   11   13   15

D. *Complex Ideational Material*

The only response required is either agreement or disagreement. Both questions for each numbered item must be answered correctly to receive credit. One repetition of each question is permitted.

1. Will a board sink in water?
   Will a stone sink in water?

2. Is a hammer good for cutting wood?
   Can you use a hammer to pound nails?

3. Do two pounds of flour weigh more than one?
   Is one pound of flour heavier than two?

4. Will water go through a good pair of rubber boots?
   Will a good pair of rubber boots keep water out?

"I am going to read you a short story and then I will ask you some questions about it. Are you ready?" (Read at a normal rate.)

Mr. Jones had to go to New York. He decided to take a train. His wife drove him to the station but on the way they had a flat tire. However, they arrived at the station just in time for him to catch the train.

5. Did Mr. Jones miss his train?
   Did he get to the station on time?

6. Was Mr. Jones going to New York?
   Was he on his way home from New York?

"I am going to read another paragraph. Are you ready?"
A soldier tried to cash a check in a bank near his camp. The teller, firm but sympathetic, said, "You will have to have identification from some of your friends from the camp." The discouraged soldier answered, "But I don't have any friends in camp—I'm the bugler."

7. Was the soldier's check cashed at once?
   Did the teller object to cashing the check?

8. Did the soldier have a friend with him?
   Did the soldier have trouble finding friends?

(10)

"I will read another one. Are you ready?"

A customer walked into a hotel carrying a coil of rope in one hand and a suitcase in the other. The hotel clerk asked, "Pardon me, sir, but will you tell me what the rope is for?"
"Yes," responded the man, "that's my fire escape!"
"I'm sorry, sir," said the clerk, "but all guests carrying their own fire escapes must pay in advance."

9. Was the customer carrying a suitcase in each hand?
   Was he carrying something unusual in one hand?

10. Did the clerk trust this guest?
    Was the clerk suspicious of this guest?

"I am going to read one more paragraph. Listen carefully."

The lion cub is born with a deep-seated hunting instinct. One cub will stalk and pounce on another with the same eagerness and thrill exhibited by a kitten. During the year and a half of cubhood this play develops into a hunting and killing technique. Skill comes through long practice, imitation of the old lions and obedience to warning growls of the mother.

11. Does this paragraph tell how to hunt lions?
    Does it tell how lions learn to hunt?

12. Does this paragraph say lions are skillful killers from the time they are born?
    Does it say lions need practice before they can kill their prey?

Score number correct: 0   1   2   3   4   5   6   7   8   9   10   11   12

III. ORAL EXPRESSION

A. *Oral Agility*

1. *Nonverbal agility:* Have the patient carry out the following rapidly repeated mouth movements as well as he can, after you demonstrate and describe the movement.
Count the number of full alternations carried out in 5 seconds.

2. *Verbal agility:* Have the patient repeat the following words as rapidly as he can, while you time the number of repetitions for 5 seconds. Any assistance which helps patient to produce the desired word initially is permitted.*
Use printed words on Card 4.

Action Required	Number of times in 5″	
	2 points	1 point
a. Purse lips, release	8	4–7
b. Open and close mouth	10	6–9
c. Retract lips, release	8	4–7
d. Tongue to alternate corners of mouth	8	4–7
e. Protrude and retract tongue	8	4–7
f. Tongue to upper and lower teeth	7	3–6

Raw Score: 0   1   2   3   4   5   6
           7   8   9 10 11 12

Test Words	Number of times in 5″	
	2 points	1 point
a. Mama, mama . . . etc.	9	3–8
b. Tip-top, tip-top	6	2–5
c. Fifty-fifty, fifty-fifty	5	2–4
d. Thanks, thanks	9	3–8
e. Huckleberry	7	3–6
f. Baseball player, Baseball player	5	2–4
g. Caterpillar	7	3–6

Raw Score: 0   1   2   3   4   5   6   7
               8   9 10 11 12 13 14

*If patient cannot get started on *one or two items at the most*, either because of perseveration or paraphasic substitution, eliminate items and prorate score. If more than two items are unscoreable, do not enter total score.

Coding of Paraphasia Columns

Paraphasic errors in single words.

1. *Neologistic distortion*—more than half of the sounds produced are extraneous to the desired word. This term applies only to responses which are spoken as a unit with some fluency of articulation. It does not apply to sounds produced by subjects groping for the correct articulatory position. Latter responses would simply be scored as failures or as severely distorted in articulation if the word is recognizable.

2. *Literal paraphasia*—response contains sounds or syllables which have slipped out of sequence, have been deleted or are entirely extraneous to the desired response, but more than half of the response corresponds to more than half of the required word.

3. *Verbal paraphasia*—substitution of an inappropriate word during the effort to say something specific.

Paraphasic errors in connected speech.

4. *Other*—this category applies to a number of types of paraphasia involving more than a single word and to some nonparaphasic responses. Examiner should write in an abbreviation of a category rather than use a checkmark only.

> *enj*—extended neologistic jargon
> *eej*—extended English jargon
> *irrel*—irrelevant speech
> *cl*—circumlocution

B. *Automatized Sequences*

Have patient recite each of the following four series, giving him assistance with the first word, if necessary. Provide further assistance as needed, but discontinue a series when patient fails with four successive words. Record assistance given by circling the word; cross out words omitted by patient. Allow 0, 1 or 2 points, as indicated.

ARTICULATION					1 point	2 points	PARAPHASIA			
Normal	Stiff	Distorted	Fail				Neologistic Distortion	Literal	Verbal	Other
				1. *Days of the week:*						
•••	•••	•••	•••	Sun. Mon. Tues.			•••	•••	•••	•••
•••	•••	•••	•••	Wed. Thur. Fri. Sat.	4 consecutive	all	•••	•••	•••	•••
				2. *Months of the year:*						
•••	•••	•••	•••	Jan. Feb. Mar. April			•••	•••	•••	•••
•••	•••	•••	•••	May June July Aug.			•••	•••	•••	•••
•••	•••	•••	•••	Sept. Oct. Nov. Dec.	5 consecutive	all	•••	•••	•••	•••
				3. *Counting to 21:*						
•••	•••	•••	•••	1 2 3 4 5 6 7 8 9			•••	•••	•••	•••
•••	•••	•••	•••	10 11 12 13 14 15 16			•••	•••	•••	•••
•••	•••	•••	•••	17 18 19 20 21	8 consecutive	all	•••	•••	•••	•••
				4. *Alphabet:*						
•••	•••	•••	•••	a b c d e f g h			•••	•••	•••	•••
•••	•••	•••	•••	i j k l m n o p q			•••	•••	•••	•••
•••	•••	•••	•••	r s t u v w x y z	7 consecutive	all	•••	•••	•••	•••
				Raw Score: 0 1 2 3 4 5 6 7 8						

C. *Recitation, Singing and Rhythm*

Instruct patient to complete the line for the following rhymes. Words in parentheses may be given as additional cues, if necessary. Use a natural or slightly exaggerated inflection to encourage completion of the rhyme. If patient fails, or is not familiar with the material, attempt other memorized or automatized matter, such as the Lord's Prayer, the Pledge of Allegiance, etc. Circle qualitative ratings below.

1. *Reciting:*

Jack and Jill (went) .... There was an old woman who lived in a shoe, (she had) ....

Baa, Baa, black sheep (have) ...

My country ('tis) ....
(Sweet) ....
(Of thee) ....

2. *Singing:* After recitation of "My Country 'Tis of Thee," have patient sing this or any other song with which he is familiar.

3. *Rhythm:* Examiner taps out the following rhythms on the desk in continuous fashion (6 times) until the patient demonstrates that he can or cannot repeat tempo.

⌣ ′ ⌣ ′ (repeat) (as in: "along, along")
′ ⌣ ⌣ ′ ⌣ ⌣ (repeat) (as in: "Longfellow")
⌣ ′ ′ ⌣ ′ ′ (repeat) (as in: "a long time")
′ ⌣ ⌣ ′ ′ , ′ ′ (as in: "Shave and a haircut, two bits")

RATINGS: *Reciting*   *Singing*   *Rhythm*
                                      (Melody)

2 = Good
1 = Impaired
0 = Failed

D. *Repetition of Words*

Have patient repeat each of the following words. One repetition by examiner is permitted when it appears that this may help, or when it is requested. For credit, all syllables must be in their proper order, although distortion of individual sound elements is permitted, provided it is in keeping with patient's general articulation difficulty and that the word is recognizable.

| ARTICULATION | | | | | Neolo-gistic | PARAPHASIA | | |
Normal	Stiff	Distorted	Fail			Literal	Verbal	Other
				what				
				chair				
				hammock				
				purple				
				brown				
				W				
				fifteen				
				1776				
				emphasize				
				Methodist Episcopal				

Raw Score: 0   1   2   3   4   5   6   7   8   9   10

(16)

E. *Repeating Phrases*

Have patient repeat the following phrases. Alternate between columns 1 and 2.
On patient's request, a single repetition of the entire test phrase is permitted
without loss of credit.

ARTICULATION						PARAPHASIA			
Normal	Stiff	Distorted	Fail	1. *High Probability*	2. *Low Probability*	Neologistic Distortion	Literal	Verbal	Other
				a. You know how.					
					a. The vat leaks.				
				b. Down to earth.					
					b. Limes are sour.				
				c. I got home from work.					
					c. The spy fled to Greece.				
				d. You should not tell her.					
					d. Pry the tin lid off.				
				e. Go ahead and do it if possible.					
					e. The Chinese fan had a rare emerald.				
				f. Near the table in the dining room.					
					f. The barn swallow captured a plump worm.				
				g. They heard him speak on the radio last night.					
					g. The lawyer's closing argument convinced him.				
				h. I stopped at his front door and rang the bell.					
					h. The phantom soared across the foggy heath.				

Raw Score: 1) 0 1 2 3 4 5 6 7 8
2) 0 1 2 3 4 5 6 7 8

F. *Word-reading*

Have the patient read the words, one at a time, from test Card 5. Check approximate lag between your pointing to the word and the patient's adequate response. Assist as required, but give no credit for responses obtained with help.

| ARTICULATION | | | | Test Words | Approximate response lag | | | | PARAPHASIA | | | |
Normal	Stiff	Distorted	Fail		0–3″ 3 points	3–10″ 2 points	10–30″ 1 point	Fail 0	Neol. Dist.	Literal	Verbal	Other
				chair								
				circle								
				hammock								
				triangle								
				fifteen								
				purple								
				seven-twenty-one								
				dripping								
				brown								
				smoking								

Raw Score: 0   3   6   9   12   15   18   21   24   27   30

G. *Responsive Naming*

Have patient supply the one-word responses required by the stimulus questions. Check approximate lag

| ARTICULATION | | | | Question | Approximate response lag | | | | PARAPHASIA | | | |
Normal	Stiff	Distorted	Fail		0–3″ 3 points	3–10″ 2 points	10–30″ 1 point	Fail 0	Neol. Dist.	Literal	Verbal	Other
				What do we tell time with?								
				What do you do with a razor?								
				What do you do with soap?								
				What do you do with a pencil?								
				What do we cut paper with?								
				What color is grass?								
				What do we light a cigarette with?								
				How many things in a dozen?								
				What color is coal?								
				Where do you go to buy medicine?								

Raw Score: 0   3   6   9   12   15   18   21   24   27   30

(18)

H. *Visual Confrontation Naming*

Have the patient name each item in the order listed as you point to it on Cards 2 and 3. Assist, if necessary, to preserve rapport, but do not credit responses so obtained. Check under column which indicated appropriate lag in giving response, and score accordingly. Articulation and paraphasia should be rated wherever possible.

ARTICULATION					Approximate response lag				PARAPHASIA			
Normal	Stiff	Distorted	Fail	Test Items	0–3″ 3 points	3–10″ 2 points	10–30″ 1 point	Fail 0	Neologistic Distortion	Literal	Verbal	Other
				Objects:								
				chair								
				key								
				glove								
				feather								
				hammock								
				cactus								
				Letters:								
				H								
				T								
				R								
				L								
				S								
				G								
				Geometric Forms:								
				square								
				triangle								
				Actions:								
				running								
				sleeping								
				drinking ·								
				smoking								
				falling								
				dripping								
				Numbers: 7								
				15								
				700								
				1936								
				42								
				7000								
				Colors:								
				red								
				brown								
				pink								
				blue								
				gray								
				purple								
				Body parts:								
				ear								
				shoulder								
				elbow								

Raw Score: 0 15 25 35 45 55 65 75 85 95 105

J. Body-part Naming

ARTICULATION					Approximate response lag				PARAPHASIA			
Normal	Stiff	Distorted	Fail		0–3″ 3 points	3–10″ 2 points	10–30″ 1 point	Fail 0	Neologistic Distortion	Literal	Verbal	Other
				ear								
				nose								
				shoulder								
				ankle								
				wrist								
				thumb								
				elbow								
				eyebrow								
				knuckles								
				shin								

Raw Score: 0   3   6   9   12   15   18   21   24   27   30

K. Animal-naming (Fluency in Controlled Association)

Instruct the patient: "I want to see how many different animals you can call to mind and name for about a minute, while I count them. Any animals will do; they can be from the farm, the jungle, the ocean or house pets. For instance you can start with dog." Start timing from this point and continue for a minute and a half. Score is based on the most productive consecutive 60 seconds. Record verbatim below.

First 15″   15–30″   30–45″   45–60″   60–75″   75–90″

Raw Score: 0–2   3–5   6–8   9–12   13–15   16–19

(20)

L. *Oral Sentence-reading*

Have the patient read the following sentences aloud from test Cards 6 and 7. Indicate by marking on this record any assistance given, omissions, substitutions, etc. One point credit is allowed for each completely correct sentence.

	Correct 1 point	Fail
You know how.		
Down to earth.		
I got home from work.		
Near the table in the dining room.		
They heard him speak on the radio last night.		
Limes are sour.		
The spy fled to Greece.		
The barn swallow captured a plump worm.		
The lawyer's closing argument convinced him.		
The phantom soared across the foggy heath.		

Raw Score: 0 1 2 3 4 5 6 7 8 9 10

(21)

IV. UNDERSTANDING WRITTEN LANGUAGE

A. *Symbol and Word Discrimination*

Point to the model letter or word on Cards 8 and 9 and have the patient locate the correct corresponding word or letter in the row beneath it.

on _____	dog _____
G _____	B _____
H _____	who _____
was_____	F _____
K _____	pal _____

Raw Score: 0   1   2   3   4   5   6   7   8   9   10

B. *Phonetic Association*

1. *Word recognition:*

Have patient point out the written word on Cards 10 and 11 corresponding to the one you give orally. The patient should be guided to the correct line on the test card. Use the following eight oral test words.

ship _____	puppy _____
pond _____	drizzle _____
book _____	hollow _____
with _____	explode _____

Raw Score: 0   1   2   3   4   5   6   7   8

2. *Comprehension of oral spelling:*

Spell the following words for the patient and have him orally identify the spelled word.

N-O	B-R-O-W-N
M-A-N	E-L-B-O-W
G-I-R-L	F-I-F-T-E-E-N
W-H-I-P	W-H-I-S-K-E-Y

Raw Score: 0   1   2   3   4   5   6   7   8

C. *Word-picture Matching*

Assorted objects, colors, etc.   Using Cards 2 and 3, and Card 5, have patient pick out appropriate picture for each word shown him.   ("Which of these pictures is this word?")   Discourage patients from reading aloud.

chair	_____	purple	_____
circle	_____	seven-twenty-one	_____
hammock	_____	dripping	_____
triangle	_____	brown	_____
fifteen	_____	smoking	_____

Raw Score: 0   1   2   3   4   5   6   7   8   9   10

D. *Reading Sentences and Paragraphs*

Patient is presented with Cards 12, 13, 14, 15 and 16 successively.   Patient indicates his selection on the card and the examiner underlines the choice in the test booklet.   Assistance may be given in the two examples, but not in the test proper.

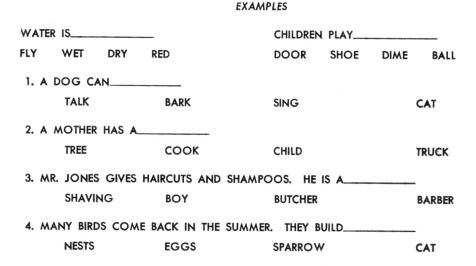

EXAMPLES

WATER IS_____   CHILDREN PLAY_____

FLY   WET   DRY   RED   DOOR   SHOE   DIME   BALL

1. A DOG CAN_____
   TALK   BARK   SING   CAT

2. A MOTHER HAS A_____
   TREE   COOK   CHILD   TRUCK

3. MR. JONES GIVES HAIRCUTS AND SHAMPOOS.   HE IS A_____
   SHAVING   BOY   BUTCHER   BARBER

4. MANY BIRDS COME BACK IN THE SUMMER.   THEY BUILD_____
   NESTS   EGGS   SPARROW   CAT

5. SCHOOLS AND ROADS COST MONEY. WE ALL PAY FOR THEM THROUGH_____

    HOUSES   COUNTRY   TAXES   POLICE

6. ARTISTS ARE PEOPLE WHO MAKE BEAUTIFUL PAINTINGS OR STATUES. ANOTHER KIND OF ARTIST IS A_____

    PICTURE   MUSICIAN   LIBRARY   SOLDIER

7. ALUMINUM WAS ONCE VERY COSTLY TO REFINE. NOW, ELECTRICITY HAS SOLVED THE REFINING PROBLEM, AND ALUMINUM HAS BECOME_____

    VERY STRONG   MUCH CHEAPER   A MINER   ELECTRONIC

8. THE CONNECTION BETWEEN SANITATION AND DISEASE BECAME CLEAR WHEN PASTEUR SHOWED THAT FOOD WOULD NOT DECAY IF GERMS WERE KILLED BY HEAT AND THEN SEALED OUT. STERILIZATION BY HEAT IS A RESULT OF_____

    SANITATION   GOOD FOOD   PASTEUR'S DISCOVERY   GERMS

9. FAVORITISM USED TO BE THE RULE IN CIVIL SERVICE, AND MANY JOBS PAID MORE THAN THEY WERE WORTH. CIVIL SERVICE REFORM HAS RESULTED IN CLASSIFYING POSITIONS ACCORDING TO THEIR DUTIES AND RESPONSIBILITIES. THE AIM OF CIVIL SERVICE CLASSIFICATION IS TO_____

    ACHIEVE HIGHER SALARIES   ESTABLISH FAVORITISM

    EFFECT A REDUCTION IN TAXES   ASSURE EQUAL PAY FOR EQUAL WORK

10. IN THE EARLY DAYS OF THIS COUNTRY, THE FUNCTIONS OF GOVERNMENT WERE FEW IN NUMBER. MOST OF THESE FUNCTIONS WERE CARRIED OUT BY LOCAL TOWN AND COUNTY OFFICIALS, WHILE CENTRALIZED AUTHORITY WAS DISTRUSTED. THE GROWTH OF INDUSTRY AND OF BIG CITIES HAS SO CHANGED THE SITUATION THAT THE FARMER OF TODAY IS CONCERNED WITH_____

    LOCAL AFFAIRS ABOVE ALL   THE PRICE OF LUMBER

    THE ACTIONS OF THE GOVERNMENT   THE AUTHORITY OF TOWN OFFICIALS

Raw Score: 0 1 2 3 4 5 6 7 8 9 10

V. WRITING

A. *Mechanics of Writing*

Recall and execution of writing movements. Have the patient execute the following (use top section of page 26 or unlined paper):

1. Name and address

2. If (1) is failed then print the patient's name and address on the paper and have him copy it.

3. Transcribe: Have the patient transcribe the sentence printed in the middle of page 26. (Note: Have the patient *write* directly on the page below the sentence. If patient cannot transcribe into longhand, have him copy in block printing.)

Evaluation of mechanics of writing: Rate the patient's writing ability, using the four-point scale listed here:

(3) Normal (making allowance for nonpreferred hand).

(2) Partly illegible but can form all letters.

(1) Fails to make many letters.

(0) No recognizable letters.

Mechanics Rating: _____

B. *Recall of Written Symbols*

For all writing tasks, continue on page 26 if practical or use additional sheets of unlined paper as necessary. Have the patient write the following:

1. *Serial writing*   Letters correct: _____

   alphabet (26 points)   Numbers correct: _____

   numbers through 21 (21 points) Letters plus numbers: _____

   Score

2. *Primer-level dictation.* Dictate the following:

   a. Single letters: Circle number correct:

      B–K–L–R–T   0 1 2 3 4 5

   b. Numbers:

      7–15–42–193–1865   0 1 2 3 4 5

   c. Primer words:

      GO–BOY–RUN–COME–BABY   0 1 2 3 4 5

      Total_____
      Score

THE QUICK BROWN FOX JUMPS OVER THE LAZY DOG

C. *Written Word-finding*

1. *Spelling to dictation:* Give the following words orally and ask the patient to write them. If a word is failed (spelled incorrectly or not written at all), have the patient spell the word orally and score in appropriate column; also provide anagrams—including two extraneous letters for each word.

	Written	Oral	Anagrams	
SOFT	_____	_____	_____	*Written Spelling*
BELONG	_____	_____	_____	Number correct:____
SOAP	_____	_____	_____	
FIGHT	_____	_____	_____	
UNCLE	_____	_____	_____	
LIBERTY	_____	_____	_____	Is oral spelling
THEATRE	_____	_____	_____	better than written?
PARTICULAR	_____	_____	_____	
PHYSICIAN	_____	_____	_____	Yes No
CONSCIENCE	_____	_____	_____	

Is anagram spelling
better than written?

Yes   No

2. *Written confrontation naming:* Using Cards 2 and 3, have the patient **write** the names of the following pictured items as they are presented by the examiner.

KEY	SEVEN
CHAIR	BROWN
CIRCLE	RED
SQUARE	DRINKING
FIFTEEN	SMOKING

Raw Score: 0 1 2 **3** 4 **5** 6 7 8 9 10

D. *Written Formulation*

1. *Narrative writing:* Present "Cookie Theft" picture (Card 1). "WRITE AS MUCH AS YOU CAN ABOUT WHAT YOU SEE GOING ON IN THIS PICTURE."
Allow patient roughly 2 minutes to write.

Score: (circle rating)
a. 0—No relevant writing
   1—Isolated words or very small groupings
   2—Incomplete, but relevant sentences
   3—Unduly simplified, but correct sentences
   4—Full description

2. *Sentences written to dictation:* Have the patient write these sentences after dictation by the examiner.

Score
a. SHE CAN'T SEE THEM. ____
b. THE BOY IS STEALING COOKIES. ____
c. IF HE IS NOT CAREFUL, THE STOOL WILL FALL. ____
Total for 3 sentences:____

b. Score each sentence as follows:
   0—Less than 2 words correct
   1—At least 2 words correct
   2—More than $\frac{1}{2}$ right
   3—Correct but laboriously done or paraphrased adequately
   4—Normally written

c. Rate paragraphic substitutions
   0—conspicuous
   1—minor
   2—absent

NOTES

NOTES

NOTES

NOTES